5-MINUTE

—— WORKOUTS FOR SENIORS ——

SCIATICA RELIEF

Your 4-Week Journey to Alleviate Chronic Pain. Low Impact Illustrated Exercises for Nerve Health, Freedom of Movement, and Rejuvenated Flexibility

EVELYN TURNER

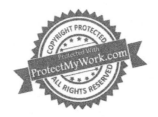

TABLE OF CONTENT

EXERCISES FLOWS

WARM-UP EXERCISES

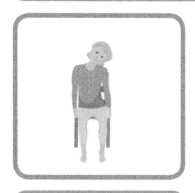

NECK TILTS
PAG. 26

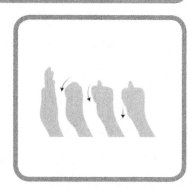

SHOULDER CIRCLES
PAG. 27

WRIST FLEXIBILITY
PAG. 28

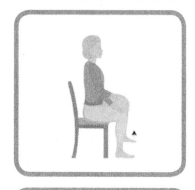

TOE TAPS
PAG. 29

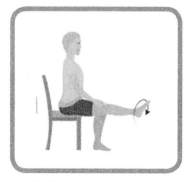

ANKLE CIRCLES
PAG.30

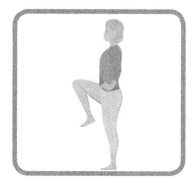

STANDING KNEE LIFTS
PAG. 31

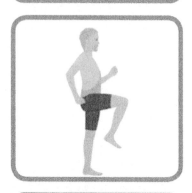

MARCHING
PAG. 32

TARGETED UPPER BODY SCIATICA RELIEF EXERCISES

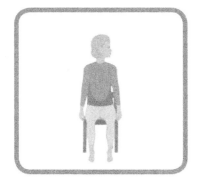

NECK ROTATION
PAG. 33

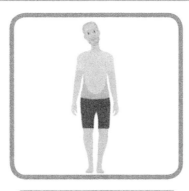

NECK FLEXION AND EXTENSION
PAG. 34

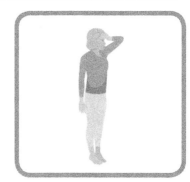

NECK RESISTANCE
PAG. 35

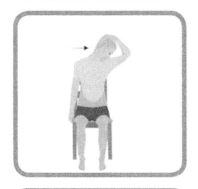

UPPER TRAP STRETCH
PAG. 36

SHOULDER BLADE SQUEEZE
PAG. 37

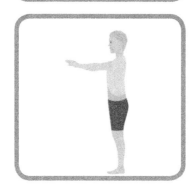

ARM RAISES
PAG. 38

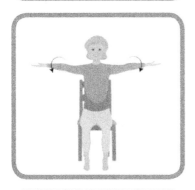

ARM CIRCLES
PAG. 39

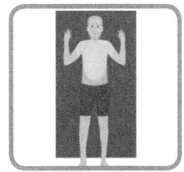

WALL ANGELS
PAG. 40

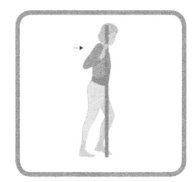

DOORWAY STRETCH
PAG. 41

TARGETED UPPER BODY SCIATICA RELIEF EXERCISES

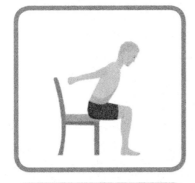

CHEST OPENER STRETCH
PAG. 42

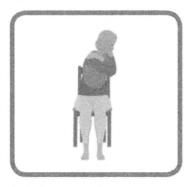

THORACIC ROTATION STRETCH
PAG. 43

TARGETED LOWER BODY SCIATICA RELIEF EXERCISES

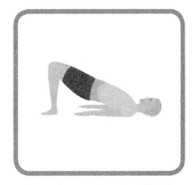

GLUTE BRIDGES
PAG. 44

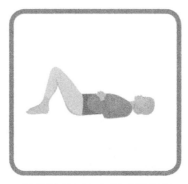

KNEE-TO-CHEST
PAG. 45

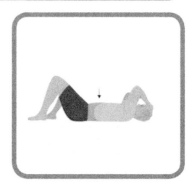

PELVIC TILTS
PAG. 46

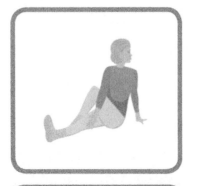

SITTING TRUNK STRETCH
PAG. 47

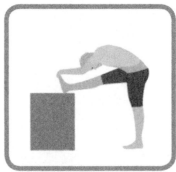

STANDING HAMSTRING STRETCH
PAG. 48

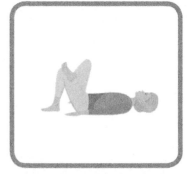

FIGURE 4 STRETCH
PAG. 49

TARGETED LOWER BODY SCIATICA RELIEF EXERCISES

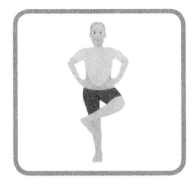

STANDING PIRIFORMIS STRETCH
PAG. 50

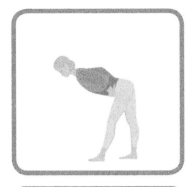

SCISSOR HAMSTRING STRETCH
PAG. 51

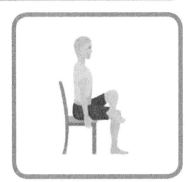

SEATED GLUTE STRETCH
PAG. 52

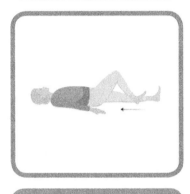

HEEL SLIDES
PAG. 53

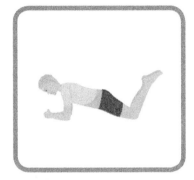

PLANK
PAG. 54

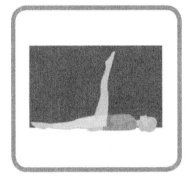

LEG RAISES
PAG. 55

TARGETED YOGA EXERCISES FOR SCIATICA RELIEF

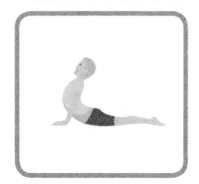

COBRA
PAG. 56

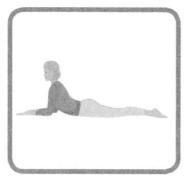

SPHINX POSE
PAG. 57

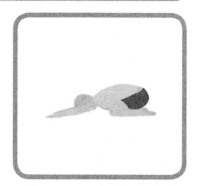

CHILD'S POSE
PAG. 58

WIND RELIEVING POSE
PAG. 59

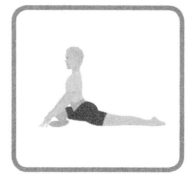

PIGEON POSE
PAG. 60

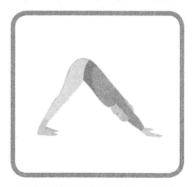

DOWNWARD FACING DOG
PAG. 61

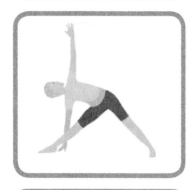

TRIANGLE POSE
PAG. 62

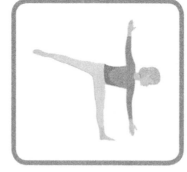

HALF MOON POSE
PAG. 63

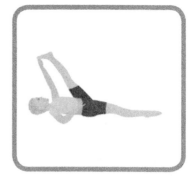

RECLINED HAND TO BIG TOE POSE
PAG. 64

TARGETED YOGA EXERCISES FOR SCIATICA RELIEF

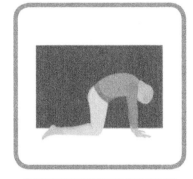

**CAT-COW STRETCH
PAG. 65**

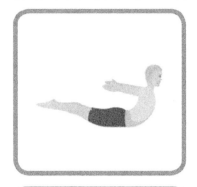

**LOCUST POSE
PAG. 66**

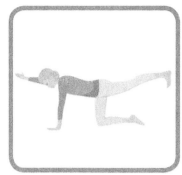

**THE BIRD-DOG POSE
PAG. 67**

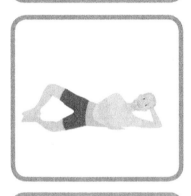

**THE CLAMSHELL
PAG. 68**

COOL DOWN EXERCISES

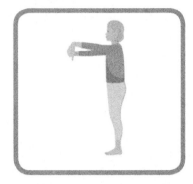

WRIST FLEXORS
PAG. 69

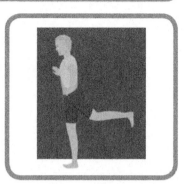

STANDING CALF STRETCH
PAG. 70

LEG SWINGS
PAG. 71

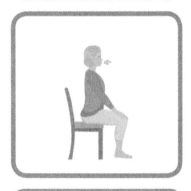

DEEP BREATHING
PAG. 72

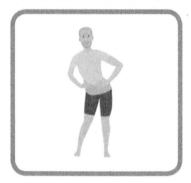

HIP CIRCLES
PAG. 73

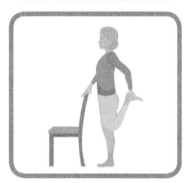

QUAD STRETCH
PAG. 74

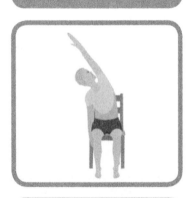

SIDE BENDS
PAG. 75

INTRODUCTION

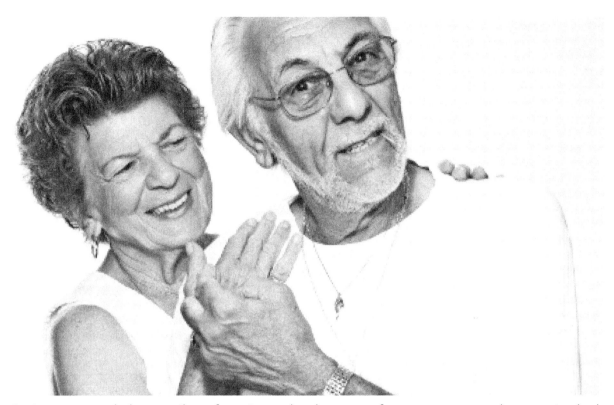

S ciatica—a word that strikes fear into the hearts of so many people, particularly seniors… That relentless, shooting pain that starts in our lower back and travels down our legs. It makes simple tasks like walking, sitting, or even getting a good night's sleep feel like monumental challenges. But of course, if you're reading this book, you already know that. I too had a bout of debilitating sciatica pain; a fact that was a major inconvenience for me.

So, allow me to introduce myself; my name is Evelyn Turner, a retired nurse who battled sciatica for some time. In the thick of things, I believed that my sciatica was a life sentence—something that would cause me discomfort and limit me through the golden years of my life. As someone who has always been reluctant to "medicate away" ailments, I chose to educate myself, looking for holistic, simple, but effective ways to manage and heal the pain I was in. And let me tell you! With the right knowledge and a bit of effort, you too can find relief and regain the freedom to enjoy your golden years to the fullest.

I wrote *5-Minute Sciatica Relief Workouts for Seniors: Your 4-Week Journey to Alleviate Chronic Pain. Low Impact Illustrated Exercises for Nerve Health, Freedom of Movement, and Rejuvenated Flexibility* because I wanted to share this holistic information with you. I am absolutely thrilled that you've picked up this book, and I can't wait to take you on a journey toward a life free from the grip of sciatica pain.

Whether you're a senior yourself or caring for a beloved elder, *5-Minute Sciatica Relief Workouts for Seniors* will introduce you to the incredible power of sciatica relief exercises and how these exercises can transform your life. And because I've experienced this journey firsthand, I can tell you just how well these exercises work. But, before I get into the details of what these exercises are and how they can transform your life, allow me to introduce you to three remarkable seniors who turned their lives around by incorporating the very exercises you're about to get started with.

Grace, at 72 years young, is a vibrant soul with a passion for dancing that has spanned her entire life. Whenever Grace spoke of her dancing days, I could really see the passion in her eyes, but sciatica pain had her in its grip, and some days, she found it difficult to even move, let alone dance. Her joy and passion for gliding across the dance floor were swiftly replaced by the agony of every step she took to do menial daily tasks. But Grace is a determined soul and she decided that sciatica wouldn't rob her of her passion, Grace embarked on the very journey of discovery you're on and with the help of gentle, scientifically formulated exercises, she began to feel relief from her sciatica pain. Slowly but surely, Grace began to regain her range of motion and the pain started to fade. Her dance shoes beckoning, Grace is not just dancing again; she's thriving.

I met Robert at the community center. Robert is a spry individual and at "68 years young," as he refers to his age, he had taken up golfing in his retirement. The sport had become Robert's sanctuary—the place where he could unwind and enjoy the outdoors once a week, surrounded by a community of like-minded people. But, sciatica hit him like a freight train and his beloved sport became a distant dream that he yearned for. Frustrated by his pain and with his muscles wasting away, Robert began to withdraw.

At a community meeting, I asked him where he had been and he confessed that his pain was so bad that some days he couldn't even tie his golf shoes, let alone practice his golf club-renowned backswing. Together, we tailored a program that could help senior golfers just like him regain their strength and flexibility, free from the grip of sciatica pain. It wasn't long before Robert was not only known for his backswing but also as the "stretch guy"—the person everyone came to for exercise advice to relieve their back pain. Robert Day by day, his strength and flexibility improved.

Finally, Sarah, who is my cousin, has always had the most incredible green thumb. She retired a bit before I did and it only seemed natural that she would spend retirement years tending to her garden. The happiness Sarah found in nurturing her plants was unparalleled, and to be honest, we loved to sit in her garden all year around, taking in the beauty and watching the birds who'd come to frolic among the flowers she'd planted. Perhaps it is a genetic component, but around the time that I began to feel the aching pain of sciatica, Sarah had reminisced she too was feeling the same tell-tale pain. Her sciatica was so bad at times that she could hardly bend over to pluck a weed without wincing in pain.

Like myself, Sarah was determined to keep her garden flourishing, and together, we began to practice these exercises and develop a holistic approach to healing our sciatica. Over time, the pain began to recede, and Sarah was back in her garden, hands in the soil, and a heart full of happiness, and of course, we continued to enjoy the fruits of her labor.

What we can learn from these three inspiring individuals is that age should never limit our potential for a vibrant, active life. With the right knowledge, from this book, and dedication, sciatica can be managed, and the pain need not define our senior years.

In reading this book we're going to dive deeper into the world of sciatica, exploring its causes and symptoms. I'll demystify the science behind relief exercises and provide you with carefully crafted routines that are specifically tailored for seniors.

Your journey toward a pain-free, active, and joyful life begins now so get comfy in your favorite chair, make yourself a cup of tea or coffee, and let's begin your 4-week journey to alleviate chronic pain.

Chapter 1
LIVING PAIN-FREE IN THE GOLDEN YEARS

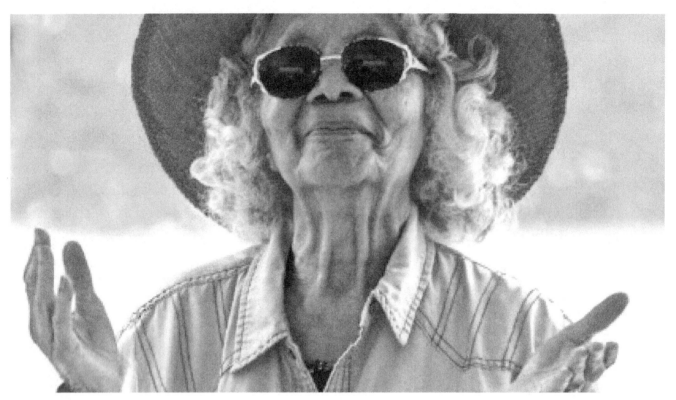

Navigating the journey of aging is like sailing through uncharted waters, it's a first for everyone, and you only turn 60 once. It's a phase of life where experiences accumulate, wisdom grows, and memories deepen. Despite this, the prospect of physical restrictions and health issues can cast a murky shadow. The importance of keeping strong, pain-free, and healthy in your later years is highlighted here—a statement that resonates strongly, especially in the context of sciatica's relentless hold.

In the realm of aging, the value of maintaining strength and vitality for yourself cannot be overstated. As the years accumulate, so do the stories etched into every wrinkle and the laughter shared with loved ones. These stories, however, are best told when the body is strong, cognizant, and capable. This synergy between age and vigor frequently translates into a quality of life defined by freedom rather than restrictions. And aging is not at all what we are led to believe, being more restricted.

It's no secret that sciatica is a powerful opponent. This unwanted visitor has a propensity for taking over even the most mundane chores. Sciatica's presence has a tendency to turn straightforward activities like sitting into conflicts, as well as more exhilarating pursuits like dancing or gardening. It is during these times that the importance of being pain-free becomes clear and dear. A pain-free life is one in which things are addressed with excitement rather than anxiety, fear, and guilt.

Consider the joy of a leisurely walk—the gentle rustle of leaves, the sunlight filtering through trees kissing your cheeks, the freedom of movement. Now, juxtapose this with the experience of walking while grappling with sciatica. Every little step becomes a strategic effort, a balancing act between the urge to move and the reality of pain. In situations like this, the vibrancy of a pain-free existence shines brightly. To move freely is to embrace the world unrestrained, to feel life's rhythm without discordant notes is something we all deserve. And the beauty of it all is the fact that it's a gift that we can give ourselves.

Furthermore, the intertwining of health and vitality in older years is a tapestry woven with threads of independence. A strong body affords autonomy—a capacity to manage daily tasks, engage in hobbies, and traverse the world with a sense of purpose. The stark contrast lies in dependence, where the lack of strength and health can tip the scales toward reliance on others, opening one up to a sense of overwhelming guilt. The existence of sciatica is a reminder of the autonomy that might dwindle if health is neglected.

Those living with sciatica, such as Grace, Robert, and Sarah, are living proof of the transformation that can occur when pain is replaced by power. Grace's return to the dance floor, Robert's improved golf swing, and Sarah's gardening all provide vivid depictions of pain-free lives. Their stories echo the larger point: that strength and freedom from pain are the foundations of a well-lived life, regardless of age. And it's wonderful to know that there are many people who have walked the path to a better life and succeeded, proving that anyone can do it.

It's important to remember that every thread counts in the vast fabric of life. Every moment spent pain-free, every activity pursued with courage, leads to a richer, more fulfilled existence. The value of staying pain-free and strong as you age is the beacon that guides the ship over tumultuous waters. Just as Martha Collins, author of "*5-Minute Sciatica Relief Workouts for Seniors*," embarked on a mission to free herself from sciatica's hold, we most certainly can all embark on a path toward a pain-free life. The relevance is profound—it is the difference between a life wasted and a life spent fully. The choice is yours.

Now, these routines are more than just boring exercises. They're your ultimate strategy to take down sciatica. You see, sciatica loves to mess with us by causing pain that starts in our lower back and shoots down our legs. But these routines, they're like the superheroes stepping in to save the day. When we target the right muscles, which make us more flexible, and help us stand tall, we're basically putting sciatica in its place.

Let's have a look at what these routines may accomplish for you. It's not simply about saying goodbye to suffering (though that's terrific). Consider walking about without that cautious tiptoe, as if you're avoiding unseen impediments. Consider bending over to tie your shoes without that cringe, as if you're performing an embarrassing ballet move. It's like saying no to pain and rediscovering the joy in everyday life.

There's more to the story than meets the eye. These practices aren't simply about getting rid of pain. They're like your secret formula for improving your overall wellness. As we get older, remaining active and feeling well becomes the ultimate objective. Consider sciatica relief exercises to be your dependable companion on this adventure. They help you stay strong, make movement easier, and serve as a gentle reminder to sciatica that it is not in charge. You are.

It's time to get real about the good stuff these routines bring for us. First off, they're totally doable, no need for fancy gyms or crazy gadgets. Nope, they're made to slide right into your daily routine. It's like setting aside a few minutes each day to open up a world of comfort and well-being. Trust me, I've been down the same road. Dealing with the same sciatica troubles. So, I get it and I can guarantee you that this will be the best investment you can ever make.

So many others serve as inspiration, faced sciatica head-on and kicked it to the curb by creating these routines. It's like she cracked the code to beat pain. And you're not in this fight alone. These routines are like your partners in this battle for a life without pain.

So, whether you're wrestling with sciatica-like a lot of us did, or just want to keep enjoying life to the fullest as you get older, these routines are your ticket. They're like a VIP pass to health and happiness. They're not just exercises; they're your way of saying, "Pain, you've had your turn. It's my time now." And who wouldn't want that?

Symptoms Associated With or Caused by Sciatic Pain

Let's dive into what it's like dealing with sciatic pain – you know, all the ins and outs of how it's playing tricks on your body. If you've walked the same path as me, you'll get it. Sciatic pain isn't just about feeling uncomfortable; it's like having your body send you mixed signals. You may have tingling sensations or your muscles may refuse to cooperate and become feeble. And what about the numbness? That's a completely different story. But wait, there's more to this saga.

This pain party has two flavors: real sciatica and sciatica-like symptoms. Sciatica is like the important guest - it's the real deal, caused by sciatic nerve pressure. Basically, it's nerve traffic congestion, and your body is most certainly not happy about it. Sciatica's cousin, sciatica-like symptoms, is another variation. It's like getting a taste of sciatica without the whole experience. You may experience tingling or discomfort, but it is not a full-fledged show. Something that is rarely discussed is the stealthy way sciatica can disrupt your restroom routine. Yes, it can cause fecal and urinary incontinence. Isn't it like putting insult to injury, right? Dealing with discomfort is one thing, but having it interfere with daily life takes it to a whole different level.

So, if you're nodding along because you know exactly what I'm talking about, you're not alone. Sciatica isn't just pain; it's like a whole bag of tricks your body didn't sign up for. But, understanding it is the first step towards heading in the right direction.

Sciatica Misconceptions

Let's talk about the sciatica misconceptions that are going about, the ones that leave you scratching your head. Believe me, I've been down that road before. Here's the skinny on what's true and what's just sciatica lore:

- Sciatica and age: Some people believe that sciatica exclusively affects the elderly. However, it does not discriminate based on age. Sciatica can strike at any age, young or old.
- One-sided affair: You've probably heard that sciatica only affects one side of the body. But, just to be clear, it has the option of affecting both sides of the body.
- The myth of rest: Here's a common misconception: resting is the remedy for sciatica. While some rest is beneficial, too much of it might actually slow down your recovery.
- Long road to recovery: Once sciatica strikes, you're in for the long haul. Not quite correct. With the proper treatment and a pinch of patience, most people begin to feel better within a few weeks.
- Exercise fear: It's a myth that sciatica prevents you from exercising. In fact, the appropriate actions can be your secret weapon against the pain.
- Just a pain problem: Sciatica isn't just about pain; it can also cause tingling, paralysis, and even interfere with your restroom routine. It might also mess with your sleep, zap your energy, and even put a dent in your social life. It is more than a bit of pain.
- Sciatica is obvious: Sometimes, the pain can be mild, and you might brush it off as just another ache. But ignoring those whispers might lead to louder shouts from your body - it might be small now, but it's a sign of something bigger.
- No pain means no sciatica: Believing that sciatica is all about pain is a bit of a misconception. It can also rear its head as a sensation of tingling, burning, or even weakness in your leg.
- It goes away on its own: Some cases of sciatica might resolve on their own, but not all of them. Ignoring persistent symptoms in hopes that they'll magically disappear can lead to further complications.

- It's only a nerve issue: The sciatic nerve, it's not always the main villain. Sometimes, muscle imbalances, spinal issues, or inflammation can contribute to the pain as well.
- One size fits all: What works for one person's sciatica might not work for another's. Each case is unique, and the right approach depends on factors like your lifestyle, overall health, and the underlying cause.

Understanding these misconceptions makes the sciatica puzzle a whole lot clearer, helping you better navigate your way to relief and wellness to live the fulfilled life you deserve.

As the years paint their brushstrokes on your life's canvas, remember that strength is the foundation upon which vitality and freedom stand. We are reminded, through the lens of sciatica, that each moment, each step, is an opportunity to demonstrate this strength, to rise above pain, and to accept the gift of living fully and without restraint in our golden years.

Chapter 2

SCIENCE AND BENEFITS OF SCIATICA RELIEF WORKOUTS

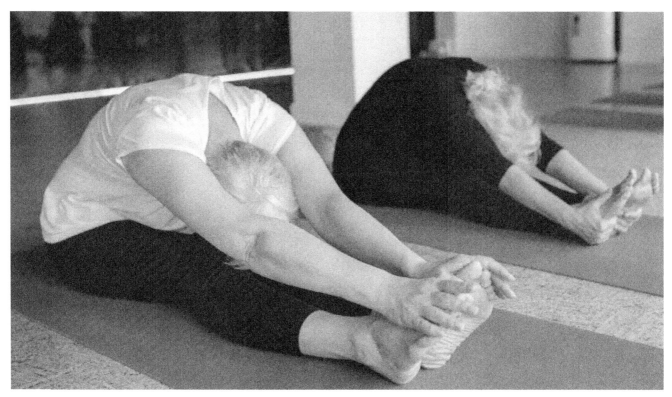

I've been right where you are now—dealing with that relentless sciatica pain that feels like it's holding you back from fully enjoying life. And if you're anything like me, you've probably spent your fair share of time wondering if there's a way to break free from its grip. But, here's your ticket to a life with less discomfort and more freedom.

This book delves into the area of sciatica relief workouts designed just for seniors like us. I understand that the concept of working out may seem scary, but trust me when I say that these aren't your regular intense gym sessions. We're talking about gentle, low-impact activities tailored to your specific needs.

See, I've been in your shoes. As a retired public school teacher, I know how important it is to stay active and enjoy the golden years. But when sciatica knocked on my door, it felt like my freedom was slipping away. Like you, I was determined not to let pain be the boss of me. So, I embarked on a journey of discovery, digging into holistic ways to manage and heal the pain that was cramping my style.

And guess what? It was successful. Those "aha" moments, those small successes mounted up, and I began to feel relieved. Slowly but steadily, I was regaining my ability to move and do the things I enjoyed without being plagued by pain. It felt like regaining control of my life. That's why I wrote this book: to share the information, exercises, and strategies that helped me. I wanted to develop a resource for seniors who are tired of letting pain dictate their lives. These sciatica cure workouts are about more than just exercises; they're about restoring your strength and mobility.

And the beauty of it all? These workouts are doable. You don't need fancy equipment or to be a fitness guru. All you need is the desire to feel better, to step into a life that's less about pain and more about possibilities. And don't worry, we're not talking hours on end – just a few minutes a day can make a world of difference.

We're going to explore how we can kick sciatica to the curb. We'll delve into the exercises, each carefully crafted to target the areas that are causing you grief. We'll learn, we'll move, and we'll show sciatica that it's no match for our determination.

The power to change your story is right here in your hands, and I'm here cheering you on every step of the way.

Sciatica Relief Workouts Can Still Be Gentle and Low-Impact and Accessible to Everyone

Let's break down the nitty-gritty of how these sciatica relief workouts are the real deal for everyone, no matter your age or fitness level. Get ready for some facts that will put a smile on your face:

- Custom-made comfort: These workouts are gentle and accommodating, recognizing that we are no longer all in our twenties. There will be no crazy acrobatics here, only movements that feel like a warm hug for your muscles and joints.
- Age is just a number: These workouts aren't exclusive to a certain age group. Whether you're 60, 70, or beyond, these exercises are here to prove that age is just a number. Your body still has plenty of vitality left, and these workouts are here to help you tap into it.
- No gym required: Forget about fancy gym memberships or intimidating equipment. These workouts are your at-home companions. All you need is a little space, maybe a mat for some cushioning, and you're ready. It's like having a personal fitness studio right in your living room.
- Baby steps: Worried about not being flexible enough? Or are you concerned that your endurance isn't what it used to be? Not a problem at all. These workouts meet you where you are and gently guide you forward.

- Low-impact: Say goodbye to those high-impact exercises, these sciatica relief workouts are all about low-impact goodness. It's still enjoyable, but much kinder to your body.
- Move without fear: Pain can make movement seem risky as if you're tiptoeing through a minefield. These workouts, on the other hand, are here to change that narrative. They're about assisting you in moving without fear and regaining faith in your own body.
- 5-minute miracles: Let's talk about time. These workouts won't demand hours of your day. In fact, just five minutes can make a world of difference. It's like finding a little oasis of relief in the midst of your day, a small investment that pays off big time.
- Real-life friendly: These routines aren't designed to turn you into a fitness guru but rather to make your daily life easier. These exercises are like little secret weapons for real-life circumstances, from getting out of bed with minimal effort to reaching the top shelf without a struggle.
- A chance to thrive: Remember the days when you felt like you could conquer the world? These workouts are a gateway straight back to that feeling. They're about helping you thrive and giving you the chance to embrace life with open arms.
- Mind-body harmony: These workouts are a symphony of mind-body harmony. They're about reconnecting with your body, about feeling more in tune with yourself.
- Minimal equipment: You won't need a basement full of equipment to get started. A chair, a mat, and maybe a resistance band, that's about it. Making it easy for you to jump in without any fuss.
- Gradual progression: Don't worry about feeling overwhelmed or pressured to perform at a certain level. These workouts are designed with a gradual progression in mind. It's all the small steps that eventually lead to big leaps in your mobility and comfort.
- Flexible schedule: Life can be busy, but that's no reason to skip these workouts. You can fit them into your schedule whenever it works for you.
- Personalized approach: These routines recognize that your path is unique. You are more than simply a face in the crowd; you are an individual with unique needs and aspirations.
- Boosts confidence: Dealing with suffering can erode your self-esteem and chip away at your confidence. These workouts are here to change that. And as you progress and feel improvements, your confidence in your body's abilities will soar.
- Strong foundation: The focus isn't just on relieving the pain but also on building a strong foundation for your body. These workouts are like the building blocks

of a sturdy structure. They strengthen your muscles, improve your posture, and enhance your overall well-being.

- Social connection: Although these workouts are appropriate for home use, you won't be traversing this journey solo. An entire community of like-minded people on the same journey as you await, with the opportunity to connect with an exercise partner if desired. Alternatively, it's an open door to engaging discussions about your workout regimen, serving as an excellent icebreaker for conversations.
- Positive mindset: The mind-body connection is powerful. These workouts don't just benefit your physical health, they also promote a positive mindset. It's like a two-in-one package deal where you're not just improving your body but also nurturing your mental wellness.
- Long-term investment: These workouts aren't a quick fix; they're a long-term investment in your health and happiness.

Benefits of Sciatica Relief Workouts for Seniors

Sciatica can really slow you down, especially as you get older. But, there's a simple way to find relief. Sciatica relief exercises can undoubtedly make a world of difference. Let's chat about why they're a game-changer.

- Easing the aches: Imagine a life with less sciatic pain. These exercises are designed to target the muscles and structures causing that pain, giving us much-needed relief.
- Getting your moves back: Sciatica often puts a kink in our mobility. But these exercises can help us get our flexibility and range of motion back. You'll find yourself moving more easily and enjoying daily activities without the discomfort.
- Living life to the fullest: Relentless sciatica pain can make life feel like a struggle. But by reducing pain and feeling more comfortable, you can replace pain with pleasure.
- Less reliance on pills: Many of us turn to medications to deal with sciatica, but they too can have their downsides. Sciatica relief exercises offer a natural alternative that might reduce our need for pills and their potential side effects.
- Keeping sciatica at bay: These exercises don't just deal with current pain; they also tackle the root causes of sciatica. By making our muscles stronger, improving our posture, and helping us stand tall, they reduce the chances of sciatica striking again.
- Sweet dreams: Sciatica often messes with our sleep. But with less pain and more comfort from these exercises, you can look forward to improved sleep.

- Boosting your mood: When we exercise, our bodies release feel-good chemicals called endorphins. It's like a natural mood booster that helps us tackle the stress and anxiety that often comes with chronic pain.
- Shedding extra pounds: Maintaining a healthy weight is vital for not only overall health in general but also for managing sciatica. These exercises can help us shed those extra pounds, taking the pressure off our sciatic nerve and reducing the chances of painful flare-ups.
- Social connections: Joining group exercise classes or activities can be a great way to meet people and stay motivated. The social aspect can provide us with a sense of community, and belonging, and provide us with meaningful interactions, which are fantastic for our mental well-being.
- Your pace, your way: These exercises can be personalized to fit your needs and abilities. You can take it easy and go at your own pace, making sure it's safe and comfortable for you.
- Embracing independence: With less pain, better mobility, and improved overall health, you can regain your independence. After all, life is all about living on your own terms.

In a nutshell, sciatica relief exercises are your secret weapon against that pesky sciatic nerve pain. Beyond just easing the pain, they're all about getting you moving better, feeling healthier, and staying happy. So, why wait? Take that first step towards relief, and let's start a journey towards a pain-free, more active, and happier life with sciatica relief exercises.

Chapter 3
ILLUSTRATED SCIATICA RELIEF EXERCISES

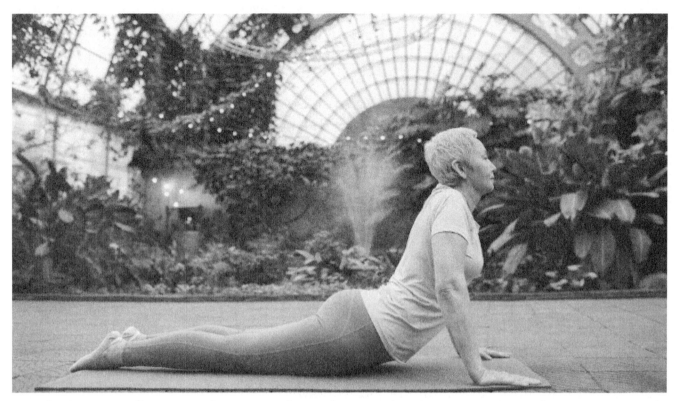

I t's time to roll up our sleeves and get down to business on our path to sciatica pain relief. This chapter is a treasure trove of 50 professionally developed exercises to assist you in finding relief. But first, let's talk about something important: warming up and cooling down.

Think of these warm-up and cool-down exercises to be your faithful protectors against injuries and post-workout stiffness. Warming up is similar to gradually waking up your body before the main event; it prepares your muscles, heart, and joints for action, making your workout safer. Now, cooling down, it's like a soothing cup of tea after a long day. It relieves muscle pain, keeps blood flowing, and can even prevent dizziness. It's a good idea to consult with your healthcare practitioner before beginning any new fitness regimen. They will assist you in tailoring your program to your specific medical conditions and physical abilities. Remember to tackle this journey to relieve sciatica pain with confidence and patience. Rather than pushing yourself too hard, concentrate on getting those motions just perfect. This method not only reduces the chance of injury but also makes the whole experience more enjoyable.

So, let's get started and work toward that wonderful alleviation from sciatica pain.

Warm-up Exercises

Warming up before exercising is more than just getting prepared. These small, repetitive efforts are crucial. Warming up has numerous health benefits, including, as previously said, supplying important nutrients and oxygen to your muscles and organs, improving blood flow, and providing joint lubrication.

This preparation benefits the body as well as the mind, emphasizing the mind-body connection. One thing is certain: An effective warm-up should stimulate your entire body, regardless of which muscle group you intend to target in your daily practice.

When you stimulate your physical systems, including your muscles, cardiovascular system, and mind, you establish the groundwork for a safe and productive workout, lowering your risk of injury.

Approach it with moderate, deliberate motions, just as you would with your regular exercises. Comfort comes first; avoid pushing yourself too hard, and remember to concentrate on your breathing to keep a consistent supply of oxygen.

Remember, what works for one person may not work for another. It's all about taking your own needs and abilities into account when engaging in a program that encourages, inspires, and ultimately benefits you.

In any new pursuit in life, it's crucial to understand that progress is a journey that demands patience.

The best part is that as time passes, you'll grow more adept in your movements, enjoying the increased strength and decreased pain and discomfort.

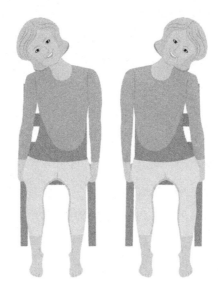

- Take a seat in a solid, sturdy chair, keep your feet hip-width apart, and placed flat on the ground.
- Maintain a straight back and relaxed shoulders.
- Keep your head straight, looking out in front of you.
- Engage your core muscles for added stability.
- Relax your arms down the sides of your body.
- Slowly and gently tilt your head to the right side as you bring your ear closer to your shoulder.
- Hold the tilted position for about 5-10 seconds.
- You should feel a gentle stretch along the side of your neck.
- Slowly return your head to the starting position.
- Now, tilt your head to the left side, bringing your ear toward the other shoulder.
- Again, hold this position for about 5-10 seconds.
- Perform 5-8 sets on each side.
- Keep the movements smooth and avoid any sudden jerks.
- Make sure your body stays in the correct posture.
- Stay in control of your movements.
- Remember to maintain a steady and relaxed breathing rhythm.
- Neck tilt exercises help improve neck flexibility and reduce tension, which is beneficial for individuals who struggle with limited neck mobility.

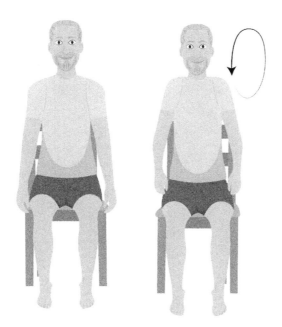

- You can do this exercise while standing upright or sitting in a sturdy chair.
- Stand with your feet hip-width apart, firmly on the ground, and keep your back straight with relaxed shoulders.
- Keep your head facing forward.
- Tighten your core muscles for better stability.
- Let your arms hang naturally by your sides.
- Inhale deeply as you slowly lift your shoulders toward your ears.
- Exhale as you roll your shoulders backward and down in a circular motion.
- Repeat this movement 8-10 times.
- After these repetitions, change direction.
- Inhale as you lift your shoulders toward your ears, then exhale as you roll them forward and down.
- Repeat this 8-10 times for each direction.
- Perform 2-3 sets.
- Keep the movements smooth and avoid any sudden jerks.
- Make sure your body stays in the correct posture.
- Stay in control of your movements.
- Remember to maintain a steady and relaxed breathing rhythm.
- If needed, perform the exercise near some support initially for added stability.
- Shoulder circle exercises are fantastic for improving your posture, increasing upper body flexibility, enhancing shoulder mobility, and reducing the risk of injury.

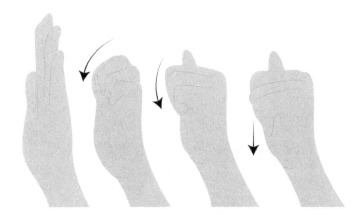

- Take a seat in a solid, sturdy chair, keep your feet hip-width apart, and placed flat on the ground.
- Maintain a straight back and relaxed shoulders.
- Keep your head straight, looking out in front of you.
- Engage your core muscles for added stability.
- Relax your arms down your sides.
- Begin with your right hand.
- Slowly and gently close your hand into a fist, curling your fingers inwards.
- Now, gently squeeze your first.
- Slowly open your hand and spread your fingers wide apart.
- You should feel a gentle stretch across the top of your hand and forearm.
- Extend your fingers as far as is comfortable without forcing them.
- Repeat this fist-to-open-hand motion 7 times.
- After completing the repetitions for one hand, switch to the other hand, and repeat.
- Perform 2-3 sets.
- Keep the movements smooth and avoid any sudden jerks.
- Make sure your body stays in the correct posture.
- Stay in control of your movements.
- Remember to maintain a steady and relaxed breathing rhythm.
- Aim to spend a total of 1-2 minutes on both hands combined.
- Wrist flexibility exercises promote mobility and reduce stiffness in the wrist joints. It also helps maintain hand function and flexibility for daily tasks.

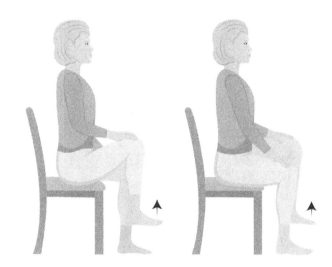

- Take a seat in a solid, sturdy chair, keep your feet hip-width apart, and place them flat on the ground.
- Maintain a straight back and relaxed shoulders.
- Keep your head straight, looking out in front of you.
- Engage your core muscles for added stability.
- Lift one foot slightly off the ground.
- Now, simply tap your toes on the floor in front of you.
- Return your foot to the starting position.
- Alternate feet and perform 10-15 taps per foot.
- Perform 2-3 sets on both sides.
- Be sure to keep your body in proper alignment.
- Maintain control over your movements.
- Remember to maintain a steady, relaxed breathing pattern.
- This exercise improves ankle mobility while also strengthening the leg muscles. It also helps to preserve lower body strength and balance, which are necessary for daily activities and fall prevention.

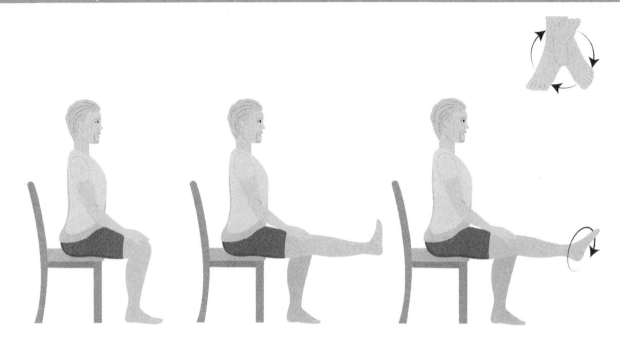

- Take a seat in a solid, sturdy chair, keep your feet hip-width apart, and placed flat on the ground.
- Maintain a straight back and relaxed shoulders.
- Keep your head straight, looking out in front of you.
- Engage your core muscles for added stability.
- Relax your arms down your sides, or hold onto your chair for extra support.
- Lift your right foot off the ground slightly, keeping the left foot firmly planted.
- Begin by gently rotating your right ankle in a clockwise direction, making circles with your foot.
- Make the circles small at first and gradually increase their size as your ankle loosens up.
- Perform 8-10 clockwise circles.
- Reverse the direction and make 8-10 counterclockwise circles with the same ankle.
- Lower the lifted foot back to the ground.
- Repeat the same sequence with your left ankle.
- Perform 2-3 sets.
- Keep the movements smooth and avoid any sudden jerks.
- Make sure your body stays in the correct posture.
- Stay in control of your movements.
- Remember to maintain a steady and relaxed breathing rhythm.
- Ankle circles improve ankle flexibility and mobility, which is beneficial for walking or standing.

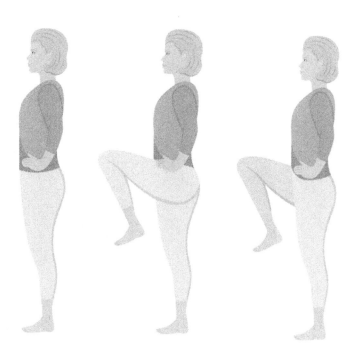

- Stand with your feet hip-width apart, firmly on the ground, and keep your back straight with relaxed shoulders.
- Keep your head facing forward.
- Tighten your core muscles for better stability.
- Place your hands on your hips or hold onto a sturdy object for support.
- Slowly lift your right knee toward your chest as high as you can.
- Hold the position for 3 seconds.
- Slowly lower your right foot back down to the ground into your starting position.
- Alternate legs and repeat this with your left knee, doing 10-15 lifts per leg.
- Keep the movements smooth and avoid any sudden jerks.
- Make sure your body stays in the correct posture.
- Stay in control of your movements.
- Remember to maintain a steady and relaxed breathing rhythm.
- Knee raises while standing enhance lower body strength, balance, and stability. This exercise also improves hip mobility, which aids in maintaining safe and confident movement in daily life and lowers the chance of falling.

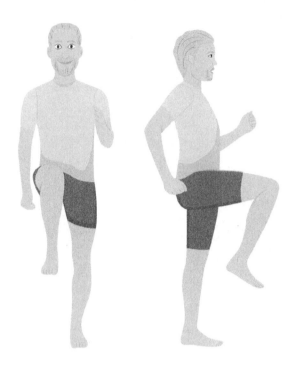

- Stand with your feet hip-width apart, firmly on the ground, and keep your back straight with relaxed shoulders.
- Keep your head facing forward.
- Tighten your core muscles for better stability.
- Place your hands on your hips to start off with, or hold onto a sturdy object for support.
- Gently and slowly swing your right knee up toward your chest.
- Immediately lower it back down to the ground, alternate legs, and lift your left knee up to your chest.
- Continue the marching motion for 1-2 minutes.
- Keep the movements smooth and avoid any sudden jerks.
- Make sure your body stays in the correct posture.
- Stay in control of your movements.
- Remember to maintain a steady and relaxed breathing rhythm.
- Warm-up marching engages the lower body and promotes circulation. It increases heart rate gradually, preparing the body for exercise. This low-impact activity enhances balance, coordination, and leg strength, vital for mobility and fall prevention.

Targeted Upper Body Sciatica Relief Exercises

From the warm-ups to the cool-downs, your body and mind are in for a treat with regular exercise. You don't have to do every exercise every day. You have the freedom to choose which muscle groups to work on and mix them up as you see fit to meet your specific needs.

Are you confused about which exercises to undertake on particular days? No worries. Chapter 4 has your back with a wonderful workout guide that will get you started on the road to pain-free living. Always prioritize quality above quantity. Dive deeply into each movement to establish that critical mind-body connection. Pay close attention to how you execute each technique, maintain a comfortable and consistent breathing rhythm, and be aware of how your body responds to each exercise. These exercises are like a blank canvas; feel free to customize them to your own needs and make incremental adjustments as you progress in your fitness journey.

Let's get started.

NECK ROTATION | *DIFFICULTY–EASY*

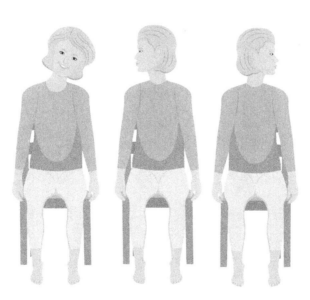

- Take a seat in a solid, sturdy chair, keep your feet hip-width apart, and placed flat on the ground.
- Maintain a straight back and relaxed shoulders.
- Keep your head straight, looking out in front of you.
- Engage your core muscles for added stability.
- Relax your arms down the sides of your body.

- Slowly and gently turn your head to the right side, trying to bring your chin towards your shoulder.
- Hold the position for 10-15 seconds, feeling a gentle stretch.
- Slowly return your head to the starting position.
- Repeat the rotation to the left side.
- Again, maintain the position for 10-15 seconds.
- Perform 3-5 sets on each side.
- Keep the movements smooth and avoid any sudden jerks.
- Make sure your body stays in the correct posture.
- Stay in control of your movements.
- Remember to maintain a steady and relaxed breathing rhythm.
- Neck rotation exercises help improve neck mobility and alleviate tension.

NECK FLEXION AND EXTENSION | *DIFFICULTY–EASY*

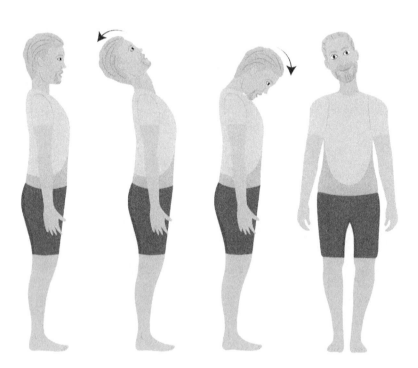

- Take a seat in a solid, sturdy chair, keep your feet hip-width apart, and place them flat on the ground.
- Maintain a straight back and relaxed shoulders.
- Keep your head straight, looking out in front of you.
- Engage your core muscles for added stability.
- Relax your arms down the sides of your body.
- For the neck flexion, slowly nod your head forward, trying to make a double chin.

- Hold the position for 5 seconds.
- Slowly return your head to the starting position.
- Now, for the neck extension, slowly tilt your head backward as if you are looking up at the ceiling.
- Hold the position for 5 seconds.
- Slowly return your head to the starting position.
- Perform 5-8 sets for both movements.
- Keep the movements smooth and avoid any sudden jerks.
- Make sure your body stays in the correct posture.
- Stay in control of your movements.
- Remember to maintain a steady and relaxed breathing rhythm.
- Neck flexion and extension exercises help improve neck mobility and alleviate tension.

NECK RESISTANCE | *DIFFICULTY–EASY*

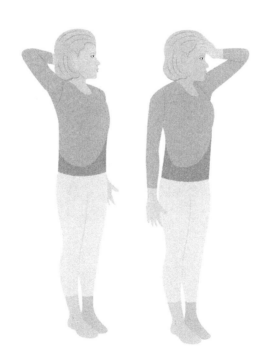

- Take a seat in a solid, sturdy chair, keep your feet hip-width apart, and place them flat on the ground.
- Maintain a straight back and relaxed shoulders.
- Keep your head straight, looking out in front of you.
- Engage your core muscles for added stability.
- Relax your arms down the sides of your body.
- Place your right hand against your forehead.

- Now gently push your head forward while at the same pushing back with your hand, resisting the forward head movement.
- Maintain this push for 5 seconds.
- Relax and return back into your starting position.
- Repeat this exercise 10 times.
- Keep the movements smooth and avoid any sudden jerks.
- Make sure your body stays in the correct posture.
- Stay in control of your movements.
- Remember to maintain a steady and relaxed breathing rhythm.
- Neck resistance exercises help strengthen the neck muscles, which facilitates improving posture and reducing tension.

UPPER TRAP STRETCH | *DIFFICULTY–EASY*

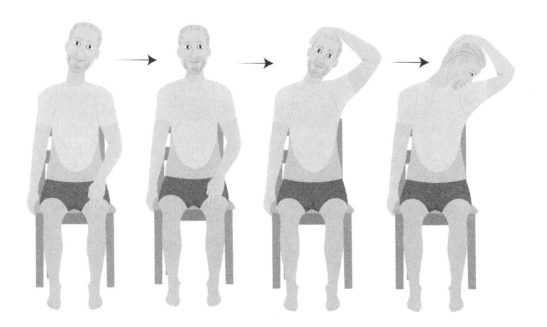

- Take a seat in a solid, sturdy chair, keep your feet hip-width apart, and place them flat on the ground.
- Maintain a straight back and relaxed shoulders.
- Keep your head straight, looking out in front of you.
- Engage your core muscles for added stability.
- Relax your arms down the sides of your body.
- Slowly and gently tilt your head to the right side, bringing your ear toward your shoulder.
- Now, gently apply pressure with your right hand to deepen the stretch.

- Maintain this position for 15-20 seconds.
- You should feel a gentle stretch along the side and back of your neck.
- Relax and return to your starting position.
- Switch to your left side and repeat.
- Perform this stretch 3-5 sets on each side.
- Keep the movements smooth and avoid any sudden jerks.
- Make sure your body stays in the correct posture.
- Stay in control of your movements.
- Remember to maintain a steady and relaxed breathing rhythm.
- Upper trap stretches are great for alleviating discomfort and tension in the neck as well as upper shoulders, reducing strain and improving posture.

SHOULDER BLADE SQUEEZE | *DIFFICULTY–EASY*

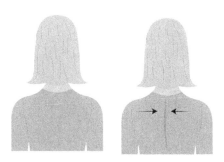

- Take a seat in a solid, sturdy chair, keep your feet hip-width apart, and place them flat on the ground.
- Maintain a straight back and relaxed shoulders.
- Keep your head straight, looking out in front of you.
- Engage your core muscles for added stability.
- Relax your arms down the sides of your body.
- Squeeze your shoulder blades together, imagining you are trying to hold a pen between them.
- Maintain this position for 5 seconds.
- Relax and release your shoulder blades as you return to your starting position.
- Repeat this squeeze 10 times.
- Keep the movements smooth and avoid any sudden jerks.
- Make sure your body stays in the correct posture.
- Stay in control of your movements.
- Remember to maintain a steady and relaxed breathing rhythm.
- Shoulder blade squeezes strengthen the muscles between the shoulder blades which helps reduce upper body tension as well as improves posture.

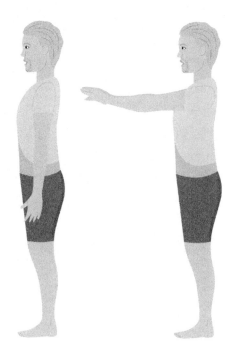

- Take a seat in a solid, sturdy chair, keep your feet hip-width apart, and place them flat on the ground.
- Maintain a straight back and relaxed shoulders.
- Keep your head straight, looking out in front of you.
- Engage your core muscles for added stability.
- Relax your arms down the sides of your body.
- Raise both arms forward and upward up to shoulder height, stretching them straight out in front of you.
- Hold this position for 5 seconds.
- Slowly lower your arms back into the starting position.
- Repeat this movement 10 times.
- Keep the movements smooth and avoid any sudden jerks.
- Make sure your body stays in the correct posture.
- Stay in control of your movements.
- Remember to maintain a steady and relaxed breathing rhythm.
- Arm raises are great for alleviating tension and improving posture.

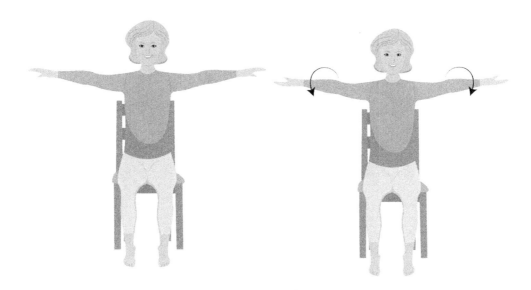

- Take a seat in a solid, sturdy chair, keep your feet hip-width apart, and place them flat on the ground.
- Maintain a straight back and relaxed shoulders.
- Keep your head straight, looking out in front of you.
- Engage your core muscles for added stability.
- Relax your arms down the sides of your body.
- Slowly extend your arms straight out to the sides.
- Begin making small circles with your arms.
- Gradually increase the size of the circles.
- After about 10 seconds, reverse the direction of the circles.
- Continue circling for a total of 30 seconds.
- Keep the movements smooth and avoid any sudden jerks.
- Make sure your body stays in the correct posture.
- Stay in control of your movements.
- Remember to maintain a steady and relaxed breathing rhythm.
- Arm circles improve shoulder mobility and posture, as well as alleviate tension.

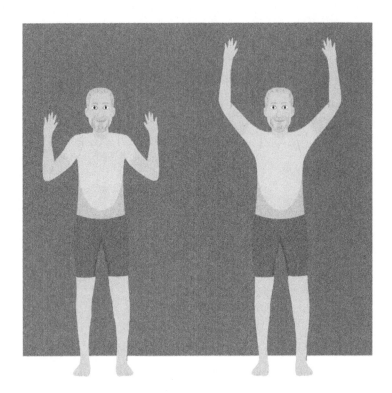

- Stand with your back against a wall.
- Keep your feet hip-width apart, placed flat and firmly on the ground.
- Maintain a straight back and relaxed shoulders.
- Keep your head straight, looking out in front of you.
- Engage your core muscles for added stability.
- Relax your arms down the sides of your body.
- Keeping your elbows bent at 90 degrees, start by slowly raising your arms to shoulder height as you slide them up along the wall.
- Continue sliding your arms upward as far as comfortable for you.
- Slide them back down into your starting position and relax.
- Perform 10-15 repetitions of this movement.
- Perform 2-3 sets.
- Keep the movements smooth and avoid any sudden jerks.
- Make sure your body stays in the correct posture.
- Stay in control of your movements.
- Remember to maintain a steady and relaxed breathing rhythm.
- Wall angels are great for alleviating upper body tension, and improving shoulder mobility as well as posture.

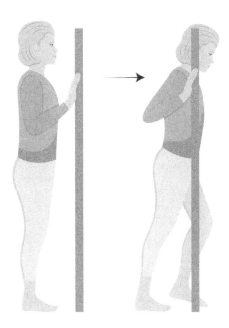

- Stand in a doorway with your feet hip-width apart, placed flat and firmly on the ground.
- Maintain a straight back and relaxed shoulders.
- Keep your head straight, looking out in front of you.
- Engage your core muscles for added stability.
- Relax your arms down the sides of your body.
- Place your hands on the doorframe at shoulder height, with your elbows bent.
- Step one foot forward and gently lean your body into the doorway, feeling a stretch in your chest and shoulders.
- Hold the stretch for 20-30 seconds.
- Switch legs and repeat.
- Perform 2-3 sets on each leg.
- Keep the movements smooth and avoid any sudden jerks.
- Make sure your body stays in the correct posture.
- Stay in control of your movements.
- Remember to maintain a steady and relaxed breathing rhythm.
- Doorway stretches are great for alleviating upper body tension and improving shoulder mobility as well as posture.

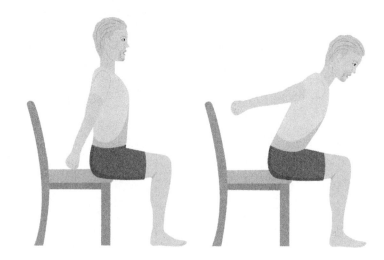

- Take a seat in a solid, sturdy chair, keep your feet hip-width apart, and place them flat on the ground.
- Maintain a straight back and relaxed shoulders.
- Keep your head straight, looking out in front of you.
- Engage your core muscles for added stability.
- Relax your arms down the sides of your body.
- Slowly clasp your hands behind your back.
- With your clasped hands, slowly start to lift your arms upward toward the ceiling.
- Lift them as high as you can until you experience a stretching sensation in your arms.
- Hold this position for 20-30 seconds.
- Slowly bring your arms back down into your starting position and relax.
- Repeat 2-3 times.
- Keep the movements smooth and avoid any sudden jerks.
- Make sure your body stays in the correct posture.
- Stay in control of your movements.
- Remember to maintain a steady and relaxed breathing rhythm.
- Chest opener stretches are great for alleviating upper body tension and improving shoulder mobility as well as posture.

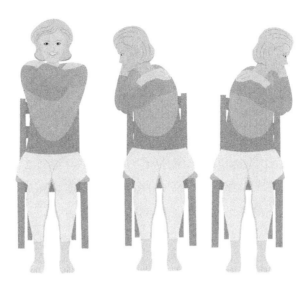

- Take a seat in a solid, sturdy chair, keep your feet hip-width apart, and place them flat on the ground.
- Maintain a straight back and relaxed shoulders.
- Keep your head straight, looking out in front of you.
- Engage your core muscles for added stability.
- Relax your arms down the sides of your body.
- Slowly bring your arms up and cross them over your chest, as if you are hugging yourself.
- Slowly rotate your upper body to the right side.
- Hold that position for 5 seconds as you feel a stretching sensation in your upper back.
- Rotate your body to the left side.
- Again, hold the position for 5 seconds.
- Perform 10 rotations on each side.
- Keep the movements smooth and avoid any sudden jerks.
- Make sure your body stays in the correct posture.
- Stay in control of your movements.
- Remember to maintain a steady and relaxed breathing rhythm.
- Thoracic rotations are great for alleviating upper body tension and improving shoulder mobility as well as posture.

Targeted Lower-Body Sciatica Relief Exercises

Let's get started with some lower-body workouts. It's the same as keeping an eye on your posture and being attentive to your approach in any training regimen.

Working out your entire body is the key to complete wellness. It's similar to keeping a well-oiled machine in good working order. But here's the golden rule: if you ever feel any discomfort or pain during your exercises, don't be too hard on yourself. It's okay to hit pause, take a breather, and then get back to it. In fact, it's better to be cautious and make gradual progress. Rushing into things can lead to injuries or stiffness that might slow down your fitness journey. So, remember to take it one step at a time, listen to your body, and give it the attention it needs.

GLUTE BRIDGES | *DIFFICULTY–EASY TO MEDIUM*

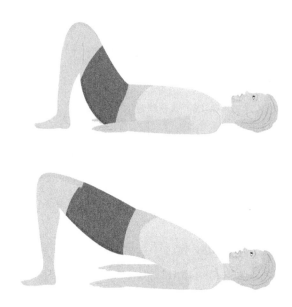

- Begin by lying flat on your back on a comfortable surface.
- Bend your legs so that your knees are pointing upwards and your feet are planted flat and firmly on the ground shoulder-width apart.
- Maintain a straight back and relaxed shoulders.
- Keep your head straight, looking out in front of you.
- Engage your core muscles for added stability.
- Push into your heels and lift your hips until your body forms a straight line from your knees to your shoulders.
- Hold the position for 5 seconds, depending on your comfort level.
- Gently lower your hips to the floor into your starting position.
- Aim for 8-10 sets initially, and gradually increase to multiple sets as it becomes more comfortable.

- Keep the movements smooth and avoid any sudden jerks.
- Make sure your body stays in the correct posture.
- Stay in control of your movements.
- Remember to maintain a steady and relaxed breathing rhythm.
- Glute bridges are great for strengthening the glute muscles, alleviating pain and discomfort, enhancing posture, and improving hip stability.

KNEE-TO-CHEST | *DIFFICULTY– EASY*

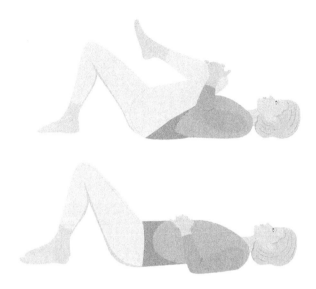

- Begin by lying flat on your back on a comfortable surface.
- Bend your legs so that your knees are pointing upwards and your feet are planted flat and firmly on the ground shoulder-width apart.
- Maintain a straight back and relaxed shoulders.
- Keep your head straight, looking out in front of you.
- Engage your core muscles for added stability.
- Bring your right knee to your chest while leaving your left foot resting on the floor.
- Hold the knee to your chest for up to 30 seconds or however long is comfortable.
- Slowly release the leg and repeat the process with the left leg.
- Perform 3 sets on each leg.
- As a variant, bring both legs to your chest and hold them for 30 seconds.
- Keep the movements smooth and avoid any sudden jerks.
- Make sure your body stays in the correct posture.
- Stay in control of your movements.
- Remember to maintain a steady and relaxed breathing rhythm.
- Knee-to-chest exercises relax the muscles, enhance circulation, relieve pain and discomfort, and improve flexibility.

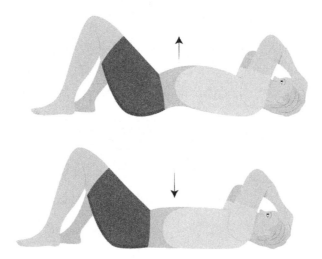

- Begin by lying flat on your back on a comfortable surface.
- Bend your legs so that your knees are pointing upwards and your feet are planted flat and firmly on the ground shoulder-width apart.
- Maintain a straight back and relaxed shoulders.
- Keep your head straight, looking out in front of you.
- Engage your core muscles for added stability and press your back into the floor.
- Tilt your hips and pelvis slightly upward.
- Holding for 5 seconds.
- Release back into your starting position and relax.
- Start with about 10 sets and gradually increase over time.
- Keep the movements smooth and avoid any sudden jerks.
- Make sure your body stays in the correct posture.
- Stay in control of your movements.
- Remember to maintain a steady and relaxed breathing rhythm.
- Pelvic tilts enhance lower back strength and stability, alleviating discomfort and improving core support. It promotes better posture and spinal alignment.

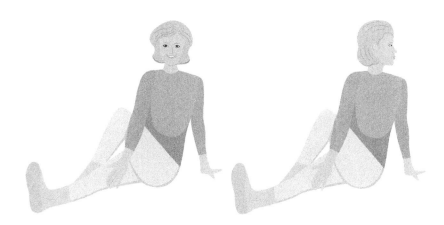

- Sit on the ground with legs straight making sure your toes are facing upward.
- Maintain a straight back and relaxed shoulders.
- Keep your head straight, looking out in front of you.
- Engage your core muscles for added stability.
- Bend your right knee, cross it over your left leg, and place it outside your left leg by the knee.
- Put your left elbow on the outside of your right knee as you gently twist toward the right.
- Hold this position for 20–30 seconds.
- Switch sides.
- Perform 2–3 sets on each side.
- Keep the movements smooth and avoid any sudden jerks.
- Make sure your body stays in the correct posture.
- Stay in control of your movements.
- Remember to maintain a steady and relaxed breathing rhythm.
- Sitting trunk stretches enhance trunk flexibility, ease lower back tension, maintain as well as improve spinal mobility, and promote better posture.

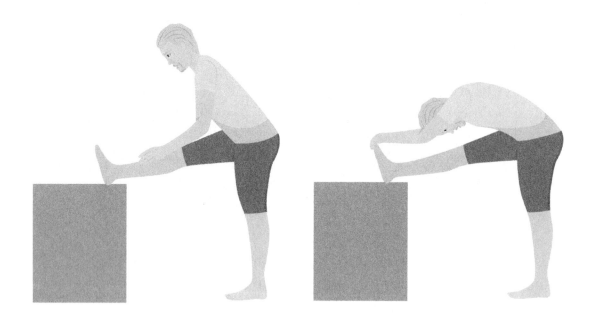

- Start off by standing with your feet placed flat and firmly on the ground, hip-width apart.
- Maintain a straight back and relaxed shoulders.
- Keep your head straight, looking out in front of you.
- Engage your core muscles for added stability.
- Place your hands on your hips or you can leave them hanging down your sides.
- You can hold onto something, such as a chair if extra balance and support are required.
- Place your right foot on something low and steady, such as a box, the seat of a sturdy chair, or even just a step.
- Keep your right leg straight.
- Flex your right foot with your toes pointed upward.
- Bend slightly forward at the hips, lowering your torso toward the leg to engage the hamstring.
- Bend down comfortably without overstretching or causing discomfort.
- Hold the position for up to 30 seconds or as long as comfortable.
- Gently release and repeat with the other leg.
- Repetitions: Aim for 2-3 sets on each leg.
- Keep the movements smooth and avoid any sudden jerks.
- Make sure your body stays in the correct posture.

- Stay in control of your movements.
- Remember to maintain a steady and relaxed breathing rhythm.
- The Standing Hamstring Stretch enhances hamstring flexibility, contributing to improved leg mobility. It also promotes flexibility in the lower back and may help reduce stiffness in the legs and lower back region.

FIGURE 4 STRETCH | *DIFFICULTY–EASY TO MEDIUM*

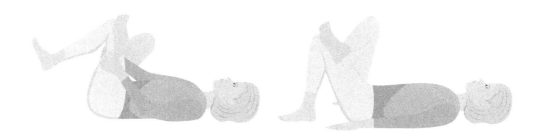

- Begin by lying flat on your back on a comfortable surface.
- Bend your legs so that your knees are pointing upwards and your feet are planted flat and firmly on the ground shoulder-width apart.
- Maintain a straight back and relaxed shoulders.
- Keep your head straight, looking out in front of you.
- Engage your core muscles for added stability and press your back into the floor.
- Cross your right foot over your left thigh.
- Move your legs up toward your torso.
- Hold the position for 5-10 seconds.
- Repeat the stretch on the other side by crossing your left foot over your right thigh.
- Perform 2-3 sets.
- Keep the movements smooth and avoid any sudden jerks.
- Make sure your body stays in the correct posture.
- Stay in control of your movements.
- Remember to maintain a steady and relaxed breathing rhythm.
- The Figure 4 Stretch is excellent for opening the hips and relieving tension in the hip area. It can help alleviate discomfort related to sciatic nerve pain. Importantly, it should be performed gently, allowing gravity to naturally deepen the stretch, rather than forcing it.

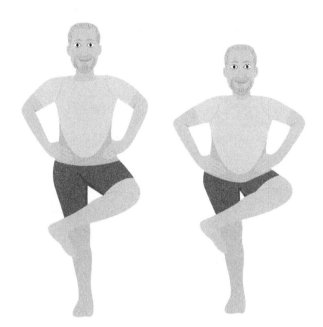

- Start off by standing with your feet placed flat and firmly on the ground, hip-width apart.
- Maintain a straight back and relaxed shoulders.
- Keep your head straight, looking out in front of you.
- Engage your core muscles for added stability.
- Place your hands on your hips or you can leave them hanging down your sides.
- You can hold onto something, such as a chair if extra balance and support are required.
- Place your right leg over the knee of your left leg, creating a "4" shape with your legs.
- Bend your standing leg while keeping your back straight and hips lowered to the ground at a 45-degree angle.
- Bend at your waist.
- Hold this stretch for 30-60 seconds.
- Switch legs and repeat the stretch on the other side.
- Perform 2-3 sets.
- Keep the movements smooth and avoid any sudden jerks.
- Make sure your body stays in the correct posture.
- Stay in control of your movements.
- Remember to maintain a steady and relaxed breathing rhythm.
- The standing piriformis stretch helps relieve sciatica pain by stretching the gluteal muscles. Regular practice can contribute to reduced discomfort in the lower back and hip area.

50

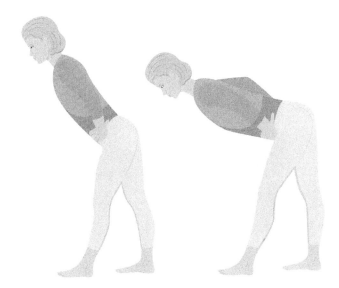

- Start off by standing with your feet placed flat and firmly on the ground, hip-width apart.
- Maintain a straight back and relaxed shoulders.
- Keep your head straight, looking out in front of you.
- Engage your core muscles for added stability.
- Place your hands on your hips for balance, or use a chair if needed.
- Move your left foot forward and place your right foot about 3 feet behind your left foot.
- Keep your hips pulled forward and shoulders pushed back, ensuring your right hip isn't farther forward than your left hip, thus keeping them aligned.
- Bend at your waist while keeping your back straight, shifting your torso slightly over your front left leg.
- Maintain your weight on your front leg during the stretch.
- Hold this position for 5-10 seconds, then switch to the opposite leg, putting your right foot in front and your left foot behind.
- Repeat the stretch 3-5 sets for each leg.
- Keep the movements smooth and avoid any sudden jerks.
- Make sure your body stays in the correct posture.
- Stay in control of your movements.
- Remember to maintain a steady and relaxed breathing rhythm.
- The "Scissor Hamstring Stretch" helps relieve sciatica pain by targeting and loosening the hamstring muscles. It can be done daily and contributes to reduced pressure on the sciatic nerve, promoting greater comfort in the lower body.

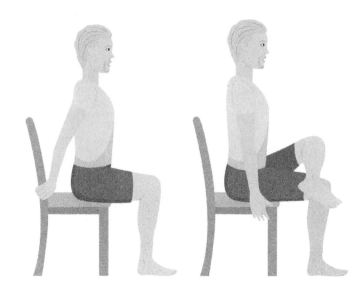

- Take a seat in a solid, sturdy chair, keep your feet hip-width apart, and place them flat on the ground.
- Maintain a straight back and relaxed shoulders.
- Keep your head straight, looking out in front of you.
- Engage your core muscles for added stability.
- Place your hands on your hips.
- Extend your legs in front of you.
- Bend your right leg, placing your right ankle on top of your left knee.
- Slowly lean forward, allowing your upper body to reach toward your right thigh.
- Hold this position for 15-30 seconds.
- Feel the stretch in your glutes and lower back.
- Repeat the stretch on the other side.
- Perform 2-3 sets on each side.
- Keep the movements smooth and avoid any sudden jerks.
- Make sure your body stays in the correct posture.
- Stay in control of your movements.
- Remember to maintain a steady and relaxed breathing rhythm.
- Seated glute stretches enhance gluteal and lower back flexibility. It helps alleviate discomfort in these areas and enhances overall comfort and mobility. Regular practice can contribute to reduced lower back tension.

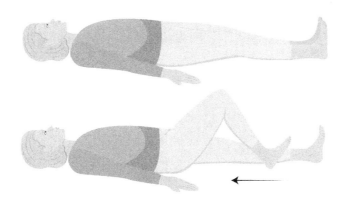

- Begin by lying flat on your back on a comfortable surface.
- Straighten your legs.
- Maintain a straight back and relaxed shoulders.
- Keep your head straight, looking out in front of you.
- Engage your core muscles for added stability.
- Pull your leg up sliding one heel along the floor toward you as you bend your knee.
- Slowly slide it back into your starting position.
- Repeat this movement for 10-15 repetitions on each leg.
- Perform 2-3 sets.
- Keep the movements smooth and avoid any sudden jerks.
- Make sure your body stays in the correct posture.
- Stay in control of your movements.
- Remember to maintain a steady and relaxed breathing rhythm.
- Heel slides are a versatile exercise that improves knee mobility, strengthens important leg muscles, aids in rehabilitation after knee surgery, relieves knee pain, and helps prevent future knee issues.

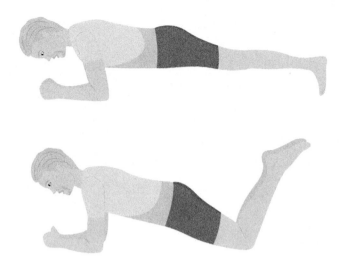

- Start off by kneeling on all fours, hands underneath your shoulders, and knees underneath your hips.
- Slowly place your forearms on the ground in front of you, lowering your body.
- Make sure your elbows are aligned with your shoulders.
- Stretch your legs out straight to the back, lifting your body off the ground.
- Keep your body in a straight line from head to heels.
- Engage your core muscles and hold this position.
- Aim to hold the plank for 20-30 seconds initially, gradually increasing the time as you get stronger.
- Perform 2-3 sets.
- Keep the movements smooth and avoid any sudden jerks.
- Make sure your body stays in the correct posture.
- Stay in control of your movements.
- Remember to maintain a steady and relaxed breathing rhythm.
- As an alternative you can lower your knees to the ground while keeping your body straight.
- Engaging in core-strengthening exercises, like planks, yields numerous benefits for seniors. These exercises promote better posture, enhance balance and stability, boost endurance, and reduce the risk of back pain, ultimately supporting spine health and overall well-being.

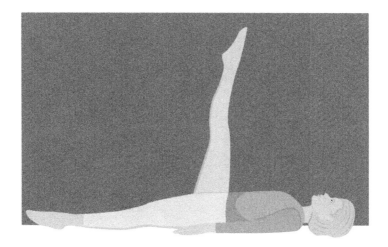

- Begin by lying flat on your back on a comfortable surface with your arms by your sides.
- Straighten your legs.
- Maintain a straight back and relaxed shoulders.
- Keep your head straight, looking out in front of you.
- Engage your core muscles for added stability.
- Slowly lift one leg while keeping it straight.
- Lift it as far as you can and hold that position for 2-3 seconds.
- Slowly lower your leg back down into the starting position.
- Repeat for 10-12 repetitions on each leg.
- Perform 2-3 sets.
- Keep the movements smooth and avoid any sudden jerks.
- Make sure your body stays in the correct posture.
- Stay in control of your movements.
- Remember to maintain a steady and relaxed breathing rhythm.
- Leg raises improve balance, enhance leg flexibility, support joint health, and strengthen core muscles for a healthy back and reduce pain.

Targeted Yoga Exercises for Sciatica Relief

I have some exciting news for you! Yoga is excellent for relieving sciatic pain, particularly from a herniated disc or piriformis syndrome. It strengthens your back muscles while stretching your hamstrings and opening up your hips, making it an ideal combination for pain relief and prevention. Remember that practice makes perfect, but if you experience any discomfort throughout your workouts, take a break and modify your program to meet your specific needs.

A study of 101 persons with chronic lower back pain was conducted in 2005 (Sherman et al., 2005). For 12 weeks, they attempted yoga, exercise, and self-care. The researchers discovered that persons who practiced yoga had the greatest improvements in their back function. These advantages persisted even after 26 weeks! Another 2015 study of 61 individuals with lower back pain, sciatica, and spinal disc abnormalities delivered rather profound results (Monro et al. 2015). Half of the individuals performed yoga for three months while the other half received standard medical care. Following the yoga session, the yoga group experienced a more significant decrease in pain and incapacity.

COBRA (BHUJANGASANA) | *DIFFICULTY–EASY TO MEDIUM*

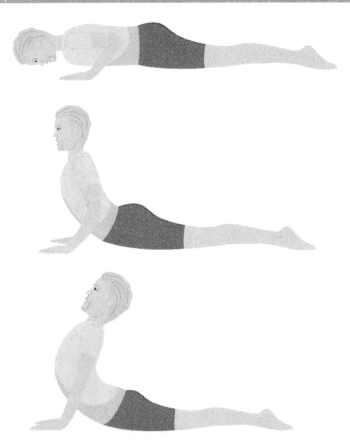

- Lie face down on a comfortable surface.
- Extend your legs, keep your feet hip-width apart, and toes pointing downward.
- Place your palms flat on the mat under your shoulders, fingers spread wide, and elbows bent and close to your body.
- Engage your pelvic floor muscles and the muscles of your lower abdomen.
- Inhale deeply and press into your palms.
- Gently lift your chest off the mat.

- Keep your pubic bone grounded and use your back muscles to lift, not pushing through your arms.
- Extend your spine as you continue to lift your chest, maintaining a slight bend in your elbows.
- Keep your shoulders relaxed.
- Tilt your head slightly upward and look forward.
- Hold the pose for 15-30 seconds, while breathing steadily.
- Exhale as you slowly release down to the mat, lowering your chest and into your starting position.
- Perform 3-5 sets.
- Keep the movements smooth and avoid any sudden jerks.
- Make sure your body stays in the correct posture.
- Stay in control of your movements.
- Remember to maintain a steady and relaxed breathing rhythm.
- Avoid straining your lower back.
- This pose should feel like a gentle backbend.
- Cobra pose helps strengthen your back muscles, improve posture, and alleviate pain by gently stretching and opening your lower back.

SPHINX POSE | *DIFFICULTY–EASY*

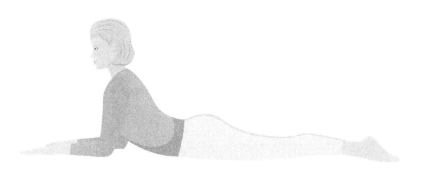

- Lie face down on a comfortable surface.
- Extend your legs, keep your feet hip-width apart, and toes pointing downward.
- Place your forearms out in front of you on the mat parallel to each other and close to your torso.
- Your elbows should be under your shoulders, forming a 90-degree angle.
- Keep your palms facing downward, fingers spread wide, and elbows bent and close to your body.
- Engage your pelvic floor muscles, and your lower abdomen, and press the tops of your feet into the mat..

- Inhale deeply and press into your palms.
- Inhale as you gently lift your upper body off the mat.
- Use your forearms for support.
- Keep your pubic bone grounded and your lower body relaxed.
- Extend your spine forward and upward to create a gentle backbend.
- Keep your shoulders relaxed.
- Look straight ahead or slightly upward.
- Hold the pose for 15-30 seconds, while breathing steadily.
- Exhale as you slowly lower your upper body back down to the mat into your starting position
- Perform 3-5 sets.
- Keep the movements smooth and avoid any sudden jerks.
- Make sure your body stays in the correct posture.
- Stay in control of your movements.
- Remember to maintain a steady and relaxed breathing rhythm.
- Avoid straining your lower back.
- The Sphinx Pose gently stretches and stimulates the spine, strengthens the core, and alleviates back pain while improving posture and enhancing lung capacity.

CHILD'S POSE | *DIFFICULTY–EASY*

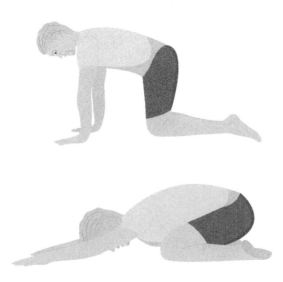

- Start off by kneeling on a comfortable surface with your knees hip-width apart.
- Bring your big toes to touch behind you, and your heels kept slightly apart.
- Sit back down on your heels and gently rest your buttocks on your feet.
- Extend your arms forward out in front of you with your palms facing downward.
- Lower your torso down towards the mat.
- Rest your forehead on the mat.

- Relax your entire body.
- Take slow, deep breaths.
- Feel the stretch along your back and spine.
- Hold the pose for at least 30 seconds.
- Gently walk your hands back towards your body to come out of the pose and back into your starting position.
- Repeat the pose for 3-5 repetitions.
- Keep the movements smooth and avoid any sudden jerks.
- Make sure your body stays in the correct posture.
- Stay in control of your movements.
- Remember to maintain a steady and relaxed breathing rhythm.
- Child's Pose helps to stretch the back, relieve stress and pain, and improve flexibility.

WIND RELIEVING POSE (PAVANAMUKTASANA) | *DIFFICULTY–EASY*

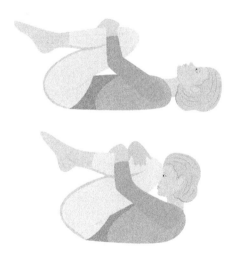

- Begin by lying flat on your back on a comfortable surface with your arms by your sides.
- Straighten your legs.
- Maintain a straight back and relaxed shoulders.
- Keep your head straight, looking out in front of you.
- Now, slowly lift both knees toward your chest as you inhale, hugging them by interlocking your fingers just below the knee.
- Be sure to keep your core engaged.
- Hold this position for 20-30 seconds while breathing steadily.
- Exhale and gently release your legs and arms back into the starting position.
- Perform 2-3 sets.

- Keep the movements smooth and avoid any sudden jerks.
- Make sure your body stays in the correct posture.
- Stay in control of your movements.
- Remember to maintain a steady and relaxed breathing rhythm.
- As a variation, you could hug one knee at a time and also curl your forward forward towards your knees for a more intensified pose.
- The Wind Relieving Pose aids digestion, releases gas and bloating, alleviates pain and discomfort, as well as stretches the lower back, and enhances flexibility.

PIGEON POSE (EKA PADA RAJAKAPOTASANA) | *DIFFICULTY—MEDIUM TO DIFFICULT*

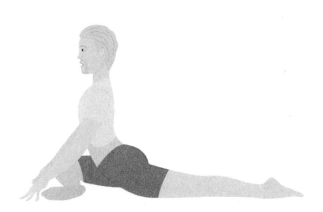

- Start off by kneeling on all fours, hands underneath your shoulders, and knees underneath your hips.
- Slide your right knee forward toward your right wrist.
- Bring your right foot across toward your left hand.
- Stretch your left leg straight out behind you.
- Ensure your hips are square and level. You can use a bolster, block, or blanket under the right buttock for support.
- Slowly and gently lower your torso toward the mat.
- Slowly walk your hands forward.
- If possible, lower your chest and forehead to the mat
- Hold the pose for 30-60 seconds, while breathing steadily.
- Press into your hands, tuck your back toes, and switch to the other side.
- Perform 2-3 sets.
- Keep the movements smooth and avoid any sudden jerks.
- Make sure your body stays in the correct posture.
- Stay in control of your movements.

- Remember to maintain a steady and relaxed breathing rhythm.
- Pigeon Pose, is excellent for hip flexibility and mobility. It also stretches the thighs, groin, and lower back, alleviating pain and tension as well as improving posture.

DOWNWARD FACING DOG (ADHO MUKHA SVANASANA) | *DIFFICULTY–EASY TO MEDIUM*

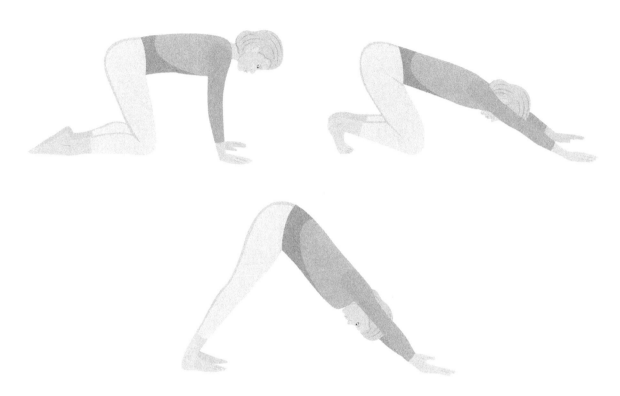

- Start off by kneeling on all fours, hands underneath your shoulders, and knees underneath your hips.
- Press your palms into the mat and spread your fingers wide apart.
- Tuck your toes under and lift your hips towards the ceiling.
- Straighten your arms and legs, forming an inverted V shape.
- Lift your hips as high as you can.
- Keep your heels grounded. Aim to press your heels toward the mat, but it's okay if they don't touch.
- Relax your head and neck, and gaze towards your knees.
- Hold the pose for 30-60 seconds, while breathing steadily.
- Slowly bend your knees and lower back into your starting position.
- Perform 2-3 sets.
- Keep the movements smooth and avoid any sudden jerks.
- Make sure your body stays in the correct posture.
- Stay in control of your movements.

- Remember to maintain a steady and relaxed breathing rhythm.
- Downward Facing Dog stretches and strengthens the entire body, including the arms, shoulders, back, and legs. This pose increases flexibility, improves posture, and relieves tension, pain, and discomfort while energizing the body and calming the mind.

TRIANGLE POSE (TRIKONASANA) | *DIFFICULTY–EASY TO MEDIUM*

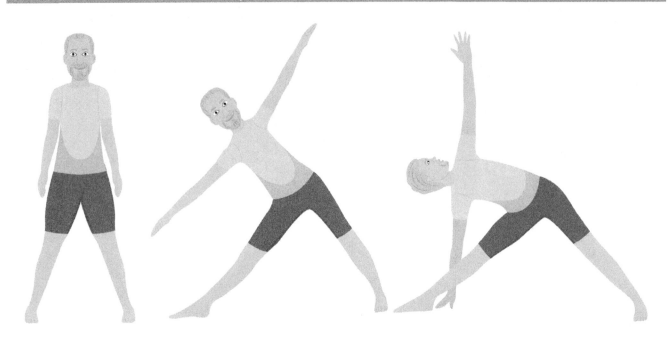

- Begin in a standing position with your feet about 3-4 feet apart and with your toes pointing forward.
- Turn your right foot 90 degrees to the right, keeping the left foot slightly turned in.
- Extend your arms parallel to the ground.
- Keep your shoulders relaxed.
- Hinge at your right hip.
- Slowly reach your right hand down toward your right ankle.
- Slowly raise your left arm upward with your fingers pointing to the ceiling.
- Turn your head to gaze up at your left fingertips.
- Hold this position for 30-60 seconds, while breathing steadily.
- Inhale as you slowly release and come back into your starting position.
- Repeat on the opposite side by turning your left foot 90 degrees to the left.
- Perform 2-3 sets.
- Keep the movements smooth and avoid any sudden jerks.
- Make sure your body stays in the correct posture.
- Stay in control of your movements.

- Remember to maintain a steady and relaxed breathing rhythm.
- Trikonasana, or Triangle Pose, stretches and strengthens the legs, hips, and torso. It improves balance, posture, and digestion while reducing stress, relieving pain and discomfort, and enhancing flexibility.

HALF MOON POSE (ARDHA CHANDRASANA) | *DIFFICULTY—MEDIUM TO DIFFICULT*

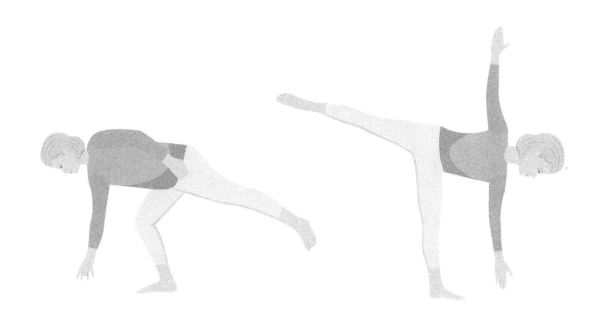

- Start off in a standing position with your feet together.
- Step your right foot back and keep it straight.
- Slowly shift your weight onto your left leg and engage your core.
- Slowly lift your right leg off the mat toward the back as you reach your left hand down toward the floor.
- Open your hips to the right and stack your left hip over your left ankle.
- Slowly extend your right arm up, aligning your shoulders.
- Look up at your right thumb.
- Maintain the pose for 20-30 seconds, while breathing steadily.
- Slowly lower your right foot and return to your starting position.
- Switch to your legs and repeat the pose on the opposite side.
- Perform 2-3 sets.
- Keep the movements smooth and avoid any sudden jerks.
- Make sure your body stays in the correct posture.
- Stay in control of your movements.
- Remember to maintain a steady and relaxed breathing rhythm.

- The Half Moon Pose improves balance, strength, and flexibility. It tones the leg muscles and engages the core while enhancing coordination. This pose also opens the chest and hips, promoting spinal alignment, overall stability, and relief from pain and discomfort.

RECLINED HAND TO BIG TOE POSE (SUPTA PADANGUSTHASANA) | *DIFFICULTY–MEDIUM TO DIFFICULT*

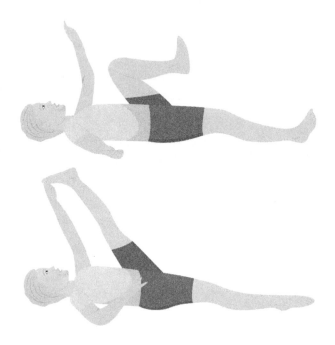

- Begin by lying flat on your back on a comfortable surface with your arms by your sides.
- Straighten your legs.
- Maintain a straight back and relaxed shoulders.
- Slowly bend your left knee and bring it toward your chest.
- Hold your left big toe with your left hand. You can also use a strap, resistance band, or belt to hold onto your big toe.
- Gently straighten your left leg upward while keeping your right leg grounded.
- Keep your foot engaged and flex it.
- Hold this position for 30-60 seconds, while breathing steadily.
- Slowly release your right leg back to the mat and into your starting position.
- Switch sides, bend your right knee, and repeat the pose on the opposite side.
- Perform 2-3 sets
- Keep the movements smooth and avoid any sudden jerks.
- Make sure your body stays in the correct posture.
- Stay in control of your movements.
- Remember to maintain a steady and relaxed breathing rhythm.

- This pose improves flexibility in the hamstrings and hip flexors. It stretches the calves and lower back, as well as relieves pain and tension, and promotes relaxation.

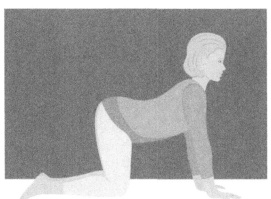 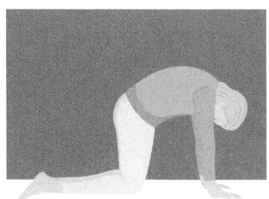

- Start off by kneeling on all fours, hands underneath your shoulders, and knees underneath your hips.
- Round your back by arching your spine upward toward the ceiling and tucking your chin towards your chest.
- Draw your belly button towards the spine.
- Arch your back in the opposite direction as you inhale, lifting your head and tailbone.
- Drop your belly towards the mat.
- Maintain an upward gaze.
- Repeat these two poses, flowing with your breath for 5 repetitions.
- Keep the movements smooth and avoid any sudden jerks.
- Make sure your body stays in the correct posture.
- Stay in control of your movements.
- Remember to maintain a steady and relaxed breathing rhythm.
- The Cat-Cow Stretch is a dynamic yoga movement that improves spine flexibility and relieves pain and tension. It enhances core strength, massages abdominal organs, and helps alleviate back pain. It also promotes better posture and reduces stress.

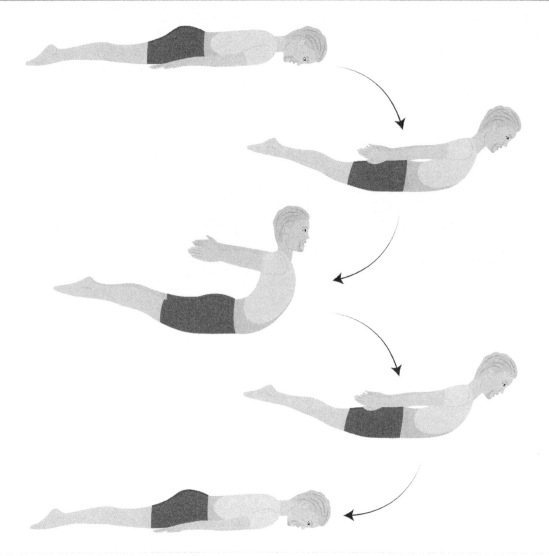

- Lie face down on a comfortable surface with your palms facing up.
- Extend your legs, keep legs and feet together, toes pointing back and downward.
- Inhale as you slowly lift your head, chest, arms, and legs all simultaneously off the mat.
- Be sure to squeeze the shoulder blades together and keep your gaze down and neck aligned.
- Hold this position for 15-30 seconds.
- Exhale and slowly release your position, lowering the mat back into your starting position.
- Perform 2-3 sets.
- Keep the movements smooth and avoid any sudden jerks.
- Make sure your body stays in the correct posture.
- Stay in control of your movements.

- Remember to maintain a steady and relaxed breathing rhythm.
- This pose strengthens the back, buttocks, and legs among other benefits. This pose also enhances spinal flexibility and relieves lower back pain.

THE BIRD-DOG POSE *(DANDAYAMANA BHARMANASANA)* | *DIFFICULTY–MEDIUM TO DIFFICULT*

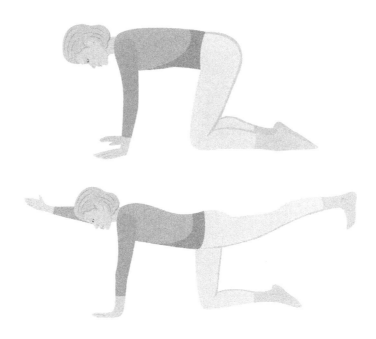

- Start off by kneeling on all fours, hands underneath your shoulders, and knees underneath your hips.
- Press your palms into the mat and spread your fingers wide apart.
- Engage your core for balance.
- Extend your right arm forward straight out in front of you and your left leg straight out backward.
- Be sure to keep them parallel to the ground.
- Hold for 10 seconds.
- Release and return to your starting position.
- Switch sides and repeat with the left arm and right leg.
- Perform 2-3 sets on each side.
- Keep the movements smooth and avoid any sudden jerks.
- Make sure your body stays in the correct posture.
- Stay in control of your movements.
- Remember to maintain a steady and relaxed breathing rhythm.
- The Bird-Dog pose strengthens the lower back, and abdominal muscles, and improves posture. It also enhances spinal stability and alleviates back pain and discomfort.

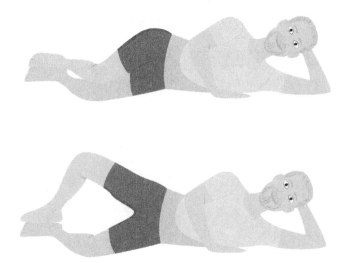

- Start off by lying on your side with your legs bent at a 90-degree angle.
- Keep your feet together with your heels touching.
- You can either rest your head on your arm or use a pillow for support.
- Inhale and slowly lift your top knee as high as comfortable, keeping your knee bent.
- Exhale and slowly lower it back down to your starting position.
- Repeat this movement for 10-15 reps before switching sides.
- Repeat the actions while lying on your opposite side.
- Perform 2-3 sets.
- Keep the movements smooth and avoid any sudden jerks.
- Make sure your body stays in the correct posture.
- Stay in control of your movements.
- Remember to maintain a steady and relaxed breathing rhythm.
- This exercise targets the hip abductors, in particular the gluteus medius. It improves hip stability, prevents hip and knee injuries, as well as enhances lower body strength and muscle balance.

Cool Down Exercises

After any given workout, how you finish significantly matters. Your body requires a gradual stop rather than a hasty one. Cooling down progressively returns your heart rate and body temperature back to their normal state, as well as reducing the discomfort of muscle stiffness. It also facilitates waste removal such as toxins, flexibility, and joint health, all of which are important for injury prevention. It's also a relaxing technique that decreases tension and provides a sense of well-being. So, following your sciatica pain reduction activities, invest a few minutes in cooling down. It will benefit both your body and mind, allowing you to stay active and free from injury and discomfort.

WRIST FLEXORS | *DIFFICULTY–EASY*

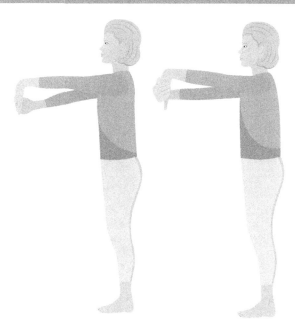

- Take a seat in a solid, sturdy chair, keep your feet hip-width apart, and place them flat on the ground.
- Maintain a straight back and relaxed shoulders.
- Keep your head straight, looking out in front of you.
- Engage your core muscles for added stability.
- Extend your right arm out in front of you with your palm facing up.
- Grip your right fingers with your left hand and gently pull them down toward the back of your wrist.
- Hold this stretch for 30 seconds.
- Next, turn your arm around so that your right palm is facing down.
- Grip the back of your right hand with your left hand and push your fingers toward your body.
- Again, hold the stretch for 30 seconds.
- Switch sides and repeat the exercise, extending your left arm out.
- Perform 2-3 sets on both sides.
- Be sure to keep your body in proper alignment.
- Maintain control over your movements.
- Remember to maintain a steady, relaxed breathing pattern.

- Regular forearm stretching reduces stiffness and muscle tightness, enhancing overall forearm flexibility. These stretches relieve discomfort and promote pain-free movement.

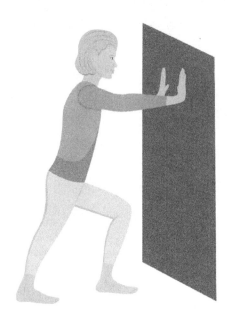

- Start off by finding sturdy support such as a wall or a chair.
- Stand with your feet placed flat and firmly on the ground, hip-width apart.
- Maintain a straight back and relaxed shoulders.
- Keep your head straight, looking out in front of you.
- Engage your core muscles for added stability.
- Step one foot back, keeping your toes pointing forward.
- Slightly bend your front knee and keep your back heel on the ground.
- Slowly lean forward, feeling the stretching sensation in your calf.
- Hold this position for 20-30 seconds.
- Release, return to your starting position, switch to the other leg, and repeat.
- Perform 2-3 sets on both sides.
- Be sure to keep your body in proper alignment.
- Maintain control over your movements.
- Remember to maintain a steady, relaxed breathing pattern.
- This stretch improves calf muscle flexibility, which reduces the risk of injury and enhances overall mobility.

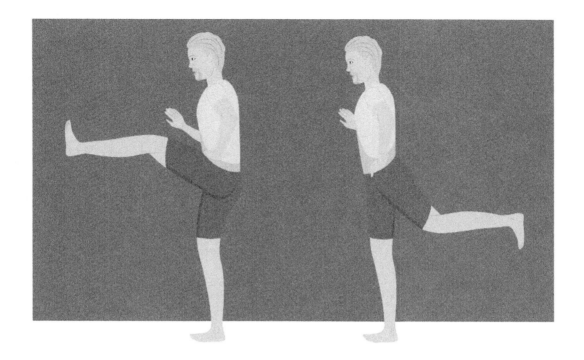

- Start off by finding sturdy support such as a wall or a chair.
- Stand with your feet placed flat and firmly on the ground, hip-width apart.
- Maintain a straight back and relaxed shoulders.
- Keep your head straight, looking out in front of you.
- Engage your core muscles for added stability.
- Start swinging your right leg forward and backward like a pendulum.
- Be sure to maintain a straight leg.
- Perform 10-15 swings before switching sides and swinging your left leg.
- Perform 2-3 sets on both sides.
- Be sure to keep your body in proper alignment.
- Maintain control over your movements.
- Remember to maintain a steady, relaxed breathing pattern.
- Leg swings improve hip and leg mobility, making daily movements like walking and climbing stairs easier. These controlled swings enhance balance and reduce the risk of trips or falls, crucial for seniors.

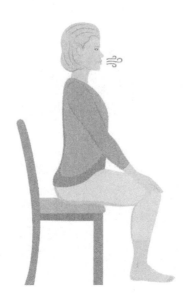

- Take a seat in a solid, sturdy chair, keep your feet hip-width apart, and place them flat on the ground.
- Maintain a straight back and relaxed shoulders.
- Keep your head straight, looking out in front of you.
- Engage your core muscles for added stability.
- Close your eyes and place your hands on your lap, or knees, or leave them hanging by your sides.
- Inhale deeply through your nose for 4 counts.
- Hold your breath for another 4 counts.
- Then, slowly exhale through your mouth for a count of 6.
- Repeat this cycle for 1-2 minutes.
- Deep breathing exercises relieve stress, promote relaxation, and aid in the management of anxiety and blood pressure. Consistent practice raises oxygen circulation, improves general well-being, and aids in stress relief and relaxation.

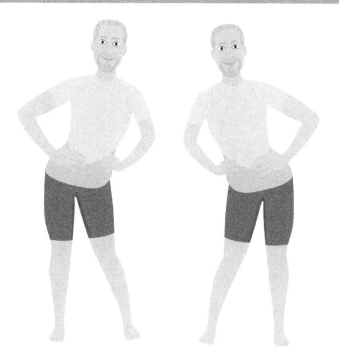

- Stand with your feet placed flat and firmly on the ground, hip-width apart.
- Maintain a straight back and relaxed shoulders.
- Keep your head straight, looking out in front of you.
- Engage your core muscles for added stability.
- Place your hands on your hips, or rest them on a stable surface.
- Slowly start rotating your hips in a clockwise, circular motion.
- Perform 10-15 circles in one direction before changing direction and rotating your hips in a counterclockwise direction.
- Perform 2-3 sets on both sides.
- Be sure to keep your body in proper alignment.
- Maintain control over your movements.
- Remember to maintain a steady, relaxed breathing pattern.
- Hip circles improve hip mobility and decrease stiffness. This exercise is excellent for improving balance, stability, and everyday movements such as getting into and out of chairs.

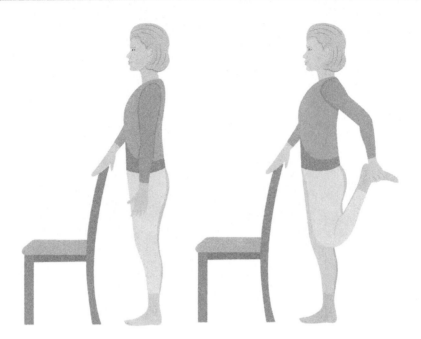

- Start off by finding sturdy support such as a wall or a chair.
- Stand with your feet placed flat and firmly on the ground, hip-width apart.
- Maintain a straight back and relaxed shoulders.
- Keep your head straight, looking out in front of you.
- Engage your core muscles for added stability.
- Hold your ankle with your hand.
- Bend your knee and bring your heel back toward your buttocks.
- Hold for 10-15 seconds.
- Release and switch to the other leg.
- Perform 2-3 sets on both sides.
- Be sure to keep your body in proper alignment.
- Maintain control over your movements.
- Remember to maintain a steady, relaxed breathing pattern.
- The quad stretch enhances flexibility and prevents muscle tightness, making daily tasks like walking and climbing stairs easier, while reducing the risk of injury.

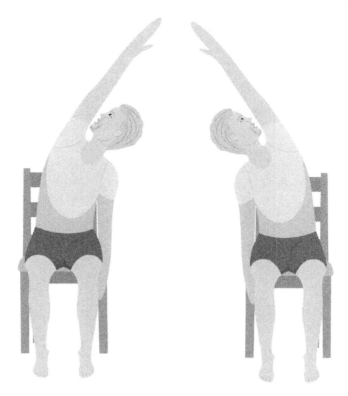

- Take a seat in a solid, sturdy chair, keep your feet hip-width apart, and place them flat on the ground.
- Maintain a straight back and relaxed shoulders.
- Keep your head straight, looking out in front of you.
- Engage your core muscles for added stability.
- Keep your arms relaxed and hanging down the sides of your body.
- Slowly lift your left arm up above your head
- With your left arm, bending at your waist, reach over the top of your head to your right.
- Maintain this position for 2 counts.
- Feel the stretch along the side of your body.
- Slowly return back to your starting position as you exhale.
- Perform 8-10 repetitions.
- Switch sides and perform the same routine, bending to the opposite side.
- Perform 2-3 sets on both sides.
- Be sure to keep your body in proper alignment.
- Maintain control over your movements.
- Remember to maintain a steady, relaxed breathing pattern.
- Avoid tilting or bending your body forward or backward.
- These stretches improve core stability, torso strength, and flexibility. It also works wonders when it comes to improving posture and balance.

Here are 50 wonderful exercises for relieving sciatica pain and stiffness, allowing you to live a more independent and pain-free life. In the following chapter, we'll take it a step further and look at an inspired workout plan to support you on your journey to healing.

Chapter 4
4-WEEK SCIATICA RELIEF WORKOUT PLAN WITH A FREE GIFT

Now that you have a diverse range of sciatica pain relief exercises at your disposal, it's time to take action. How? By exploring a straightforward, comprehensive exercise plan that will inspire you to lead the pain-free, fulfilling life you deserve.

This plan will systematically introduce all 50 sciatica pain relief exercises over four weeks. You'll find a convenient table for guidance on initial repetitions. And there's more: As you read on, you'll uncover a pleasant bonus: a special gift to help you measure your progress and celebrate your accomplishments!

Week-by-week Wall Pilates Workout Plan

Let's steer clear of becoming demotivated. Before commencing any of the exercises detailed in the workout plan, it's imperative to keep in mind the necessity of executing warm-up routines and cool-down exercises afterward. This precautionary step is crucial in mitigating the risk of potential muscle strain or injury that could render you inactive. Remember, baby steps, stay within your capabilities and needs.

WEEK 1: KICKING OFF YOUR BALANCE JOURNEY		
Day 1		
Exercise	*Page*	*Repetitions*
Neck Rotation	33	Maintain position for 10-15 seconds Perform 3-5 sets in each direction
Upper Trap Stretch	36	Maintain position for 10-15 seconds Perform 3-5 sets on each side
Sitting Trunk Stretch	47	Maintain position for 20-30 seconds Perform 2-3 sets on each side
Seated Glute Stretch	52	Maintain position for 15-30 seconds Perform 2-3 sets on each side
Sphinx Pose	57	Maintain position for 15-30 seconds Perform 3-5 sets

Day 2		
Neck Flexion and Extension	34	Maintain position for 5 seconds. Perform 5-8 sets on each side
Shoulder Blade Squeeze	37	Perform squeeze 10 times
Heel slides	53	Perform 5-10 repetitions on each leg Perform 2-3 sets
Leg Raises	55	Perform 10-12 repetitions on each leg Perform 2-3 sets
Child's Pose	58	Maintain position for 5 seconds Perform 3-5 sets
Day 3		
Neck Resistance	35	Maintain position for 5 seconds Perform 10 sets
Arm Raises	38	Maintain position for 5 seconds Perform 10 sets
Knee-to-Chest	45	Maintain position for 30 seconds Perform 3 sets on each leg
Scissor Hamstring Stretch	51	Maintain position for 5-10 seconds Perform 3-5 sets on each leg
Wind Relieving Pose	59	Maintain position for 20-30 seconds Perform 2-3 sets
Day 4		
Arm Circles	39	Circle clockwise and counterclockwise for 30 seconds
Chest Opener Stretch	42	Maintain position for 20-30 counts Perform 2-3 sets
Leg Raises	55	Perform 10-12 repetitions for each leg Perform 2-3 sets
Seated Glute Stretch	52	Maintain position for 15-30 seconds Perform 2-3 sets
Sphinx Pose	57	Maintain position for 15-30 seconds Perform 3-5 sets

Day 5		
Wall Angels	40	Perform 10-15 repetitions Perform 2-3 sets
Thoracic Rotation Stretch	43	Maintain position for 5 seconds Perform 10 rotations on each side
Knee-to-Chest	45	Maintain position for 30 seconds Perform 3 sets on each leg
Heel slides	53	Perform 5-10 repetitions on each leg Perform 2-3 sets
Child's Pose	58	Maintain position for 5 seconds Perform 3-5 sets
Day 6		
Rest		

WEEK 2: GAINING STRENGTH

Day 7

Asana/Stretch	Page	Repetitions
Doorway Stretch	41	Maintain position for 20-30 seconds Perform 2-3 sets on each leg
Shoulder Blade Squeeze	37	Perform squeeze 10 times
Pelvic Tilts	46	Maintain position for 5 seconds Perform 10 sets
Standing Hamstring Stretch	48	Maintain position for 30 seconds Perform 2-3 sets on each leg
Cobra	56	Maintain position for 15-30 seconds Perform 3-5 sets

Day 8

Chest Opener Stretch	42	Maintain position for 20-30 seconds Perform 2-3 sets
Neck Resistance	35	Maintain position for 5 seconds Perform 10 sets
Glute Bridges	44	Maintain position for 5 seconds Perform 8-10 sets
Figure 4 Stretch	49	Maintain position for 5-10 seconds Perform 2-3 sets on each leg
Downward Facing Dog	61	Maintain position for 30-60 seconds Perform 2-3 sets

Day 9

Upper Trap Stretch	36	Maintain position for 10-15 seconds Perform 3-5 sets on each side
Wall Angels	40	Perform 10-15 repetitions Perform 2-3 sets
Pelvic Tilts	46	Maintain position for 5 seconds Perform 10 sets
Knee-to-Chest	45	Maintain position for 30 seconds Perform 3 sets on each leg
Triangle Pose	62	Maintain position for 30-60 seconds Perform 2-3 sets

Day 10		
Doorway Stretch	41	Maintain position for 20-30 seconds Perform 2-3 sets on each leg
Arm Raises	38	Maintain position for 5 seconds Perform 10 sets
Figure 4 Stretch	49	Maintain position for 5-10 seconds Perform 2-3 sets on each leg
Heel slides	53	Perform 5-10 repetitions on each leg Perform 2-3 sets
Cat-Cow Stretch	65	Perform 5 sets
Day 11		
Arm Circles	39	Circle clockwise and counterclockwise for 30 seconds
Thoracic Rotation Stretch	43	Maintain position for 5 seconds Perform 10 rotations on each side
Seated Glute Stretch	52	Maintain position for 15-30 seconds Perform 2-3 sets
Scissor Hamstring Stretch	51	Maintain position for 5-10 seconds Perform 3-5 sets on each leg
The Bird-Dog Pose	67	Maintain position for 10 seconds Perform 2-3 sets on each side
Day 12		
Rest		

WEEK 3: RAMPING IT UP

Day 13

Asana/Stretch	Page	Repetitions
Doorway Stretch	41	Maintain position for 20-30 seconds Perform 2-3 sets on each leg
Arm Circles	39	Circle clockwise and counterclockwise for 30 sec.
Leg Raises	55	Perform 10-12 repetitions for each leg Perform 2-3 sets
Scissor Hamstring Stretch	51	Maintain position for 5-10 seconds Perform 3-5 sets on each leg
The Clamshell	68	Perform 10-15 repetitions for each side Perform 2-3 sets

Day 14

Neck Flexion and Extension	34	Maintain position for 5 seconds Perform 5-8 sets on each side
Figure 4 Stretch	49	Maintain position for 5-10 seconds Perform 2-3 sets on each leg
Cat-Cow Stretch	65	Perform 5 sets
Child's Pose	58	Maintain position for 5 seconds Perform 3-5 sets
Reclined Hand to Big Toe Pose	64	Maintain position for 30-60 sec. on each side Perform 2-3 sets

Day 15

Thoracic Rotation Stretch	43	Maintain position for 5 seconds Perform 10 rotations on each side
Seated Glute Stretch	52	Maintain position for 15-30 seconds Perform 2-3 sets
Standing Piriformis Stretch	50	Maintain position for 30-60 seconds on each side. Perform 2-3 sets
Half Moon Pose	63	Maintain position for 20-30 seconds on each side. Perform 2-3 sets
Pigeon Pose	60	Maintain position for 30-60 seconds on each side. Perform 2-3 sets

Day 16

Doorway Stretch	41	Maintain position for 20-30 seconds Perform 2-3 sets on each leg
Knee-to-Chest	45	Maintain position for 30 seconds Perform 3 sets on each leg
Reclined Hand to Big Toe Pose	64	Maintain position for 30-60 seconds on each side. Perform 2-3 sets
Scissor Hamstring Stretch	51	Maintain position for 5-10 seconds Perform 3-5 sets on each leg
Standing Piriformis Stretch	50	Maintain position for 30-60 seconds on each side. Perform 2-3 sets

Day 17

Upper Trap Stretch	36	Maintain position for 10-15 seconds Perform 3-5 sets on each side
Standing Hamstring Stretch	48	Maintain position for 30 seconds Perform 2-3 sets on each leg
Half Moon Pose	63	Maintain position for 20-30 seconds on each side. Perform 2-3 sets
Reclined Hand to Big Toe Pose	64	Maintain position for 30-60 seconds on each side. Perform 2-3 sets
Triangle Pose	62	Maintain position for 30-60 seconds Perform 2-3 sets

Day 18

Rest

WEEK 4: STRONG AND FLEXIBLE

Day 19

Asana/Stretch	Page	Repetitions
Doorway Stretch	41	Maintain position for 20-30 seconds Perform 2-3 sets on each leg
Glute Bridges	44	Maintain position for 5 seconds. 8-10 sets
Plank	54	Maintain position for 20-30 seconds. 2-3 sets
Locust Pose	66	Maintain position for 15-30 seconds. 2-3 sets
Pigeon Pose	60	Maintain position for 30-60 seconds on each side. Perform 2-3 sets

Day 20

Chest Opener Stretch	42	Maintain position for 20-30 counts Perform 2-3 sets
Leg Raises	55	Perform 10-12 repetitions for each leg. Perform 2-3 sets
Standing Piriformis Stretch	50	Maintain position for 30-60 seconds on each side. Perform 2-3 sets
Half Moon Pose	63	Maintain position for 20-30 seconds on each side. Perform 2-3 sets
Scissor Hamstring Stretch	51	Maintain position for 5-10 seconds Perform 3-5 sets on each leg

Day 21

Doorway Stretch	41	Maintain position for 20-30 seconds Perform 2-3 sets on each leg
Half Moon Pose	63	Maintain position for 20-30 seconds on each side. Perform 2-3 sets
Glute Bridges	44	Maintain position for 5 seconds Perform 8-10 sets
Plank	54	Maintain position for 20-30 seconds. Perform 2-3 sets
Reclined Hand to Big Toe Pose	64	Maintain position for 30-60 seconds on each side. Perform 2-3 sets

Day 22		
Standing Piriformis Stretch	50	Maintain position for 30-60 seconds on each side. Perform 2-3 sets
Pelvic Tilts	46	Maintain position for 5 seconds Perform 10 sets
Sphinx Pose	57	Maintain position for 15-30 seconds Perform 3-5 sets
Locust Pose	66	Maintain position for 15-30 seconds Perform 2-3 sets
The Bird-Dog Pose	67	Maintain position for 10 seconds Perform 2-3 sets on each side
Day 23		
Doorway Stretch	41	Maintain position for 20-30 seconds Perform 2-3 sets on each leg
Half Moon Pose	63	Maintain position for 20-30 seconds on each side. Perform 2-3 sets
Glute Bridges	44	Maintain position for 5 seconds Perform 8-10 sets
Plank	54	Maintain position for 20-30 seconds Perform 2-3 sets
The Clamshell	68	Perform 10-15 repetitions for each side Perform 2-3 sets
Day 24		
Rest		

STRETCH AND RECOVERY WEEK

Day 25

Stretch	Page	Repetitions
Neck Tilts	26	Maintain position for 5-10 seconds Perform 5-8 sets on each side
Wrist Flexibility	28	Perform 7 repetitions for each side Perform 2-3 sets
Ankle Circles	30	Perform 8-10 repetitions for each side and each direction. Perform 2-3 sets
Standing Calf Stretch	70	Maintain position for 20-30 seconds Perform 2-3 sets on each side
Deep Breathing	72	Repeat the breathing cycle for 1-2 minutes

Day 26

Shoulder Circles	27	Perform 8-10 repetitions in each direction Perform 2-3 sets
Toe Taps	29	Perform 10-15 repetitions per foot Perform 2-3 sets
Standing Knee Lifts	31	Maintain position for 3 seconds Perform 10-15 lifts on each leg
Wrist Flexors	69	Maintain position for 30 seconds Perform 2-3 sets on each side
Leg Swings	71	Perform 10-15 swings on each side Perform 2-3 sets

Day 27

Marching	32	March for 1-2 minutes
Neck Tilts	26	Maintain position for 5-10 seconds Perform 5-8 sets on each side
Hip Circles	73	Perform 10-15 repetitions in each direction Perform 2-3 sets
Quad Stretch	74	Maintain position for 10-15 seconds on each side. Perform 2-3 sets
Side Bends	75	Perform 8-10 repetitions on each side Perform 2-3 sets

Day 28		
Wrist Flexibility	28	Perform 7 repetitions for each side Perform 2-3 sets
Shoulder Circles	27	Perform 8-10 repetitions in each direction Perform 2-3 sets
Wrist Flexors	69	Maintain position for 30 seconds Perform 2-3 sets on each side
Leg Swings	71	Perform 10-15 swings on each side Perform 2-3 sets
Deep Breathing	72	Repeat the breathing cycle for 1-2 minutes
Day 29		
Marching	32	March for 1-2 minutes
Standing Knee Lifts	31	Maintain position for 3 seconds Perform 10-15 lifts on each leg
Ankle Circles	30	Perform 8-10 repetitions for each side and each direction Perform 2-3 sets
Standing Calf Stretch	70	Maintain position for 20-30 seconds Perform 2-3 sets on each side
Deep Breathing	72	Repeat the breathing cycle for 1-2 minutes
Day 30		
Rest		

Monitoring Your Progress and Celebrating Your Achievements

Have you ever started a new journey, whether it's to live a better lifestyle, acquire a new skill, or pursue your aspirations, and wondered why it's so crucial to celebrate tiny triumphs along the way?

In all honesty, tracking our goals and achievements can be tough, however, it's worth it. There are various reasons why it's challenging. And, these reasons differ from person to person. First, some of us often lack consistency. We start with enthusiasm but struggle to stick to a routine due to life's unpredictability and distractions. Setting too many goals can overwhelm us, making it hard to track progress effectively. Unrealistic goals can be discouraging, leading us to quit tracking. Clear metrics and milestones are crucial, but vague goals make tracking difficult. Fear of failure can also hold us back, as we avoid facing setbacks. Our busy lives and fading motivation add to the challenge. Ineffective tracking tools, resistance to change, and fear of accountability are all further aspects that add to these challenges and complicate matters even more for us.

But all is not lost, there is some great news. Despite these obstacles, tracking offers clarity, motivation, and a sense of accomplishment. To overcome them, set realistic goals, establish a clear tracking system, and stay disciplined. Support from friends or professionals for accountability and encouragement is another fantastic aspect to consider. At the end of the day, tracking is a powerful tool to facilitate personal growth and success.

We are often so focused on achieving our objectives that we fail to recognize and take pleasure in our accomplishments. However, celebrating accomplishments and tracking your progress is undeniably a game changer. When you accomplish something, no matter how modest, your brain releases feel-good hormones like dopamine. This makes you happy and keeps you motivated to keep going. Celebrating your successes also boosts your confidence. It demonstrates your ability, making you more willing to take on new challenges.

Monitoring your progress is like having a map for your journey. It reminds you of how far you've come and keeps you focused on your goals. This is especially helpful during difficult times since it keeps you motivated and on track. Life can be challenging at times, with many ups and downs. However, celebrating your victories acts as a protective shield against feeling deterred. You know you've overcome hurdles in the past, so you're more resilient when confronted with new ones. You get more confident in your abilities as your self-confidence rises. Mistakes are essentially lessons we can learn from.

Finally, recognizing your accomplishments keeps everything in perspective. It serves as a reminder that life is a journey, and each stride forward is something to be proud of. It encourages you to enjoy the voyage and appreciate all of the tiny and major moments. So, whether you're pursuing your aspirations, overcoming sciatic pain, or simply trying to be a better version of yourself, don't forget to celebrate your accomplishments and track your progress. Starting a new workout plan to relieve sciatic pain is an excellent opportunity for a fresh start, a new chapter. Allow me to share some exciting news with you to help you celebrate your new adventure.

You'll see a QR code directly below that you can scan to get your free, downloadable, and printable version of the *ForeverFit Progress Journal*. With this journal, you'll find your motivation, establish self-discipline, track your progress, and happily celebrate your fitness and wellness accomplishments.

This journal provides you with a wonderful opportunity to contemplate each stage of your voyage, celebrating your achievements while also observing areas where there may be potential for improvement. It serves as a valuable instrument for investigating recurring challenges and uncovering fresh insights about yourself. Once you've identified these hurdles, you can set to work on surmounting them, refining your objectives, and shifting your focus toward cultivating a robust and adaptable senior physique.

Taking all of these aspects into consideration and equipped with your personalized workout plan, the final leg of our journey entails developing self-discipline in our senior years. With this understanding, you'll be prepared through the upcoming chapter, where you'll learn how to attain a pain-free existence, reclaim your independence, and fully embrace life.

SCAN ME

Chapter 5
HOW TO BUILD SELF-DISCIPLINE AND STAY MOTIVATED

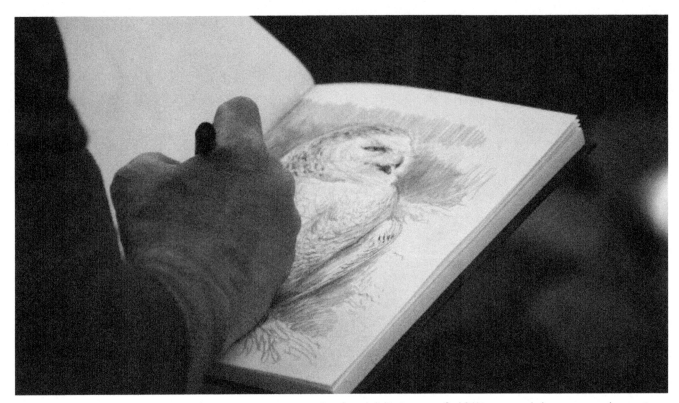

In the journey toward sciatica pain relief and living a fulfilling golden era, there's a secret weapon that can make all the difference: a growth mindset. A simple yet incredibly powerful concept. And it's something that anyone, at any age, can embrace. So, what exactly is a growth mindset, and why is it so vital, especially in the golden years of life?

Consider a mindset in which you feel that your abilities and intelligence are not fixed attributes, but can be cultivated and enhanced through time. This is exactly what a growth mindset entails. It is the concept that obstacles, setbacks, and even failures are chances for growth and learning rather than roadblocks. Consider them to be life's tiny lessons. After all, life is a series of ups and downs. For if there were just happy times, how could we enjoy them if there were no terrible moments to contrast them with?

Instead of seeing limitations, a person with a growth mindset sees possibilities and opportunities. For seniors, adopting a growth mindset can be transformative. And let me tell you, it's never too late to make healthy changes. It's a mindset that can help you navigate the challenges that often come with aging, including managing sciatica pain. This mindset helps us better embrace challenges. With age, our bodies might not be as spry as they once were, and health issues like sciatica can become more prevalent.

A growth mindset encourages seniors to embrace these challenges as opportunities for personal development. It is a mode of thinking that states, "I can learn, adapt, and find ways to alleviate this pain." A growth mentality builds resilience, which is especially important in later life. When faced with difficulty or pain, seniors with a growth mentality are more likely to weather the storm and recover. They feel that setbacks are only transitory and that they can overcome them. Seniors with a growth mentality have an insatiable quest for information. They recognize that the brain, like a muscle, improves with training. They understand that it is never too late to learn anything new, whether it be new pain treatment techniques, a new pastime, or simply staying cognitively engaged.

Believe it or not, a growth mindset can have a positive impact on physical health. Seniors who see room for growth are more inclined to exercise regularly and make healthier lifestyle choices. And this is precisely what you seek. Relieving sciatica and improving general health. Emotional resilience and well-being are directly tied to a growth mindset. Seniors who see problems as opportunities report less stress and anxiety because they are more prepared to deal with life's ups and downs. The best part of it all is that a growth mindset fosters a more positive outlook, which can lead to improved relationships with family and friends.

It's never too late to adopt a growth mindset, no matter your age or circumstances. Here are a few simple steps to get started:

- Embrace challenges: When faced with a challenge, resist the urge to see it as a roadblock. Instead, view it as an opportunity to learn and grow. Approach it with curiosity and an open mind instead of fear.
- The power of "yet": If you catch yourself saying, "I can't do this," add the word "yet" at the end. This simple addition opens the door to future growth and improvement, self-belief, motivation, and confidence.
- Love learning: Make a commitment to lifelong learning. Whether it's reading a book, taking up a new hobby, or learning about pain relief techniques, keep your mind engaged and curious. Think of the mind-body connection where a healthy mind means a healthy body and vice versa.
- Surround yourself with positivity: Seek out positive influences and surround yourself with people who support your growth mindset and your pain-free journey. Share your journey with friends and family who encourage your efforts and help keep you accountable.

It's a mindset that empowers you to take charge of your health and well-being, see opportunities where others see obstacles, and continue growing and learning throughout your senior years. It's a perspective that reminds you that it's never too late to adopt a better, more beneficial outlook on life—one that can lead to a pain-free and fulfilling senior existence.

Healthy Diet and Exercise for Sciatica Pain Relief in Seniors

Two superheroes arrive to save the day in the fight against sciatica pain alleviation and overall well-being: a good diet and frequent exercise. These two vital components of each person's lifestyle are more than just companions; they are a dynamic couple that collaborates to achieve an overall happier and healthier life. Let's look at the harmonious link between diet and exercise and how they help each other.

- Diet nourishes the body: A nutritious diet offers the fuel required to power your exercise program. When you eat a nutritious, vitamin- and mineral-rich diet, your body has the energy it needs to engage in physical exercise. Exercise can feel like an uphill battle without these vital nutrients, especially for seniors suffering from sciatica pain. A proper diet ensures that your body does not only execute but also recovers from exercises successfully.

- Weight management: A well-balanced diet and exercise plan can assist seniors in maintaining a healthy weight, which is essential when it comes to managing sciatica pain. Excess weight can put extra strain on the spine and exacerbate sciatica symptoms. Exercise burns calories, and a healthy diet helps you maintain your ideal, healthy weight, minimizing the strain on your sciatic nerve and thus alleviating pain.

- Accountability: Combining nutrition and exercise helps to establish a healthy routine and accountability. Seniors can keep on track and motivated by planning meals and workouts together, having one aspect facilitate another. Knowing that exercise and a healthy diet are linked promotes consistency in both areas.

- Exercise boosts metabolism and maintains appetite control: Regular exercise has the amazing ability to rev up your metabolism. This works wonders for weight management, an important element in sciatica pain alleviation. Exercise also helps to manage hunger, making it easier to maintain a healthy diet. The more you exercise, the more in tune your body becomes with its nutritional needs, resulting in better food choices and portion control.

- Improved sleep: Regular exercise promotes better sleep, while a healthy diet can aid in quality rest. Adequate sleep is critical for recuperation and pain management, making this power couple even more useful for seniors suffering from sciatica.

- Joint health and flexibility: Exercise, particularly low-impact activities such as yoga or swimming, can improve joint health and flexibility. Reduced inflammation in the body results in less pain and greater mobility. Combine this with an anti-inflammatory diet rich in fruits and vegetables, as well as omega-3 fatty acids found in fish, and you have a winning mix for treating sciatica pain.

- Mental well-being: Diet and exercise both have a big impact on mental health. Regular physical activity releases endorphins, which are feel-good hormones that improve your mood and reduce stress. When you're in a good mood, you're more likely to make healthy food choices, steering clear from things such as emotional binge eating. This reinforces a well-being cycle that benefits both parts of a healthier lifestyle.
- Long-term health benefits: Diet and exercise work together to help with more than just sciatica pain treatment. They minimize the risk of chronic diseases such as heart disease, diabetes, and hypertension, which are common concerns in our golden years. It's more than just being healthy, you are investing in your long-term health and well-being by adopting these behaviors.

Remember that nutrition and exercise, like your mind and body, are inseparable partners on your path to relieving sciatica pain and leading a better lifestyle as a senior. They empower one another, resulting in a synergy that leads to better overall health, pain alleviation, and a higher quality of life. Whether you want to lose weight, gain flexibility, or simply feel better, embracing both components of this powerful combination can be your ticket to a brighter and more comfortable future.

Tailoring Fitness to Your Lifestyle

Your fitness choices are quite important when it comes to sciatica pain alleviation and overall well-being in your senior years. The key to success is to choose workouts that not only address your sciatica pain but also fit in with your specific lifestyle and limits. Let's look at why it's important to choose senior workouts carefully and how to do it.

- Adaptation to physical limitations: Seniors may encounter limitations in their abilities as a result of age-related changes such as arthritis, joint stiffness, and sciatica pain. This makes senior workouts utterly important and great at the same time because of their capacity to adapt to these restrictions. Low-impact exercises, mild stretches, and flexibility-focused routines can help relieve discomfort and improve mobility without exacerbating existing problems.
- Sustainable and enjoyable: The most effective senior workouts are ones that you can maintain and enjoy. Fitness should improve your quality of life rather than become a chore. Consider activities that you truly enjoy, such as swimming, Tai Chi, stretching, light cardio, or simply taking quick walks in the park. You're more likely to persist with your workouts if you enjoy them.
- Tailored to sciatica pain relief: Sciatica discomfort necessitates a unique strategy. The importance of senior exercises in this context stems from their capacity to

target and relieve chronic pain. Gentle yoga or Pilates, which develops core muscles, can provide significant comfort by stabilizing the spine and minimizing strain on the sciatic nerve. Thus, you will notice that a lot of the exercises in this book are focused on these aspects.

- Balance and fall prevention: Seniors are frequently concerned about their balance and the prevention of falls since it is one of the biggest threats we face in our golden years. Workouts that improve balance and coordination can reduce the chance of accidents and lower fall risks. Balance exercises, chair yoga, and resistance band training can all be incorporated into your regimen to achieve this.

- Personalized fitness plans: Every senior's lifestyle and constraints are distinct because our aging journeys are all unique. This is why tailored exercise plans are so beneficial. A plan suited to your own needs and goals guarantees that you are not overexerting yourself or ignoring critical parts of your health. Consult a fitness professional to develop a regimen that is right for you.

- Social connection: Senior workouts are important for reasons other than physical health. Exercise can be a social activity that helps people connect with one another, preventing that much-dreaded isolation that is a stark reality many face in their golden years. Joining a group fitness class or walking club encourages not only physical fitness but also a sense of community and support.

- Mental well-being: Senior workouts have a significant impact on mental health. Endorphins are released as a result of regular physical activity, which improves mood and reduces stress. These advantages are especially essential for seniors suffering from sciatica pain, as a cheerful attitude can also better assist with pain management.

- Consistency over intensity: Seniors should put consistency ahead of intensity. Yes, quality over quantity as they say. While high-intensity workouts are beneficial, consistency is essential for long-term health. Choose less strenuous workouts that you can commit to on a regular basis. The importance is in developing a long-term workout program.

- Mindful recovery: I reiterate, that recovery is critical in senior workouts. Proper rest and recovery between sessions are essential to prevent injury and ensure that your body can heal and grow stronger. Make sure your workout schedule includes ample time for rest and recovery.

- Consultation with healthcare professionals: Seniors may have health conditions and medications that affect exercise choices. It is critical to consult with healthcare professionals such as your doctor or a physical therapist. They can advise you on exercises that are both safe and effective to meet your specific needs.

The importance of senior exercises cannot be emphasized. Choosing workouts that fit your lifestyle and limits is essential for sciatica pain alleviation and general wellness.

Finally, activities that are entertaining, adaptable, and personalized to your specific needs will result in a more rewarding and comfortable senior life. Senior workouts improve mental well-being, social relationships, and a good view of life, in addition to physical health.

Whether you want to relieve sciatica pain, enhance your balance, or simply live a healthy life, making wise exercise choices can make all the difference. Remember, it's never too late to start a fitness routine that works for you and improves your overall health. So, take the initial step, stick with it, and get the rewards of a pain-free and enjoyable senior life.

CONCLUSION

So we've come to the end of this book and the very start of your new pain-free journey. With your new journal and 50 excellent exercises in hand, you are more than ready to embark on your new adventure and have so much to look forward to as you strive to live your best life.

It's no secret that the road of aging is an unknown land, full of experiences, insights, and memories that deepen. However, the looming shadow of physical limitations and health difficulties remains. Staying strong, pain-free, and healthy in your senior years is entirely possible, especially in the context of sciatica. Limitations should not be associated with aging. It's about adopting a high-quality existence marked by freedom and vitality. Sciatica, a tough foe, emphasizes the value of pain-free living. A pain-free life permits you to approach life with enthusiasm rather than anxiety, fear, or guilt. Consider how a leisurely stroll, the warmth of the sun, and the freedom of mobility may all become treasured pleasures in a pain-free life. Sciatica may make every movement painful.

In our golden years, independence and autonomy are woven into the tapestry of health and energy. A healthy physique allows you to manage daily tasks, pursue interests, and stay focused on your goals. Neglecting your health can develop into reliance, which can lead to feelings of crushing guilt. Real-life examples such as Grace's return to dance, Robert's better golf swing, and Sarah's gardening demonstrate the transformational impact of pain-free living. These anecdotes emphasize that, regardless of age, strength and freedom from pain are the foundations of a well-lived life. Staying pain-free and powerful as you age helps you through life's difficulties.

I get it. The idea of working out might seem intimidating, especially when you're dealing with sciatica. But trust me when I say, these sciatica relief workouts are not your typical intense gym sessions. They are gentle, low-impact exercises that are tailor-made for folks like us. You see, I've been right where you are now. I know how important it is to stay active and make the most of our golden years. But when sciatica came knocking at my door, it felt like my freedom was slipping away, I felt robbed. However, just like you, I was determined not to let pain dictate my life's course.

In Chapter 3 you were armed with a treasure trove of 50 professionally crafted exercises, and we also discussed a couple of crucial things: warm-up and cool-down exercises. Think of warm-up and cool-down exercises as your trusted companions on this journey. Warming up gradually rouses your body, preparing your muscles, heart, and joints for activity and providing a more secure workout. Cooling down, on the other hand, is like drinking a calming cup of tea after a long day: it relieves muscle pain, keeps circulation moving, and prevents disorientation. Progress is a journey that requires patience, but as time passes, you'll notice that you're becoming more adept at your motions, with increasing strength and less pain and discomfort.

The importance of tracking your progress and celebrating your accomplishments cannot be overstated as you know by now. It's a powerful tool for personal growth and success. Despite the challenges, tracking offers clarity, motivation, and a sense of accomplishment. Setting realistic goals, establishing a clear tracking system, seeking support from friends or professionals, and staying disciplined are keys to overcoming obstacles.

Thus, as you embark on this new chapter of relieving sciatic pain and improving your overall well-being, don't forget to celebrate your accomplishments and track your progress. You're on a journey toward a pain-free existence, independence, and embracing life to the fullest, that is a whole lot to look forward to and enough to keep you motivated. To help you celebrate and stay motivated, remember to scan the QR code to access your free *ForeverFit Progress Journal*.

This journal will be your companion on this exciting adventure, providing motivation, self-discipline, progress tracking, and a deeper understanding of yourself.

As we come to the end of this book and your road toward sciatica pain treatment and a rewarding golden era, I'd like to remind you of one strong tool that can truly make a difference: a development mindset. It's a simple yet immensely powerful principle that anyone, of any age, can embrace. A growth mindset is based on the belief that your abilities and intelligence are not fixed attributes that can be developed and improved over time. It is about perceiving challenges, setbacks, and even failures as chances for growth and learning rather than impassable walls. It's a way of thinking that helps you to perceive possibilities and opportunities rather than restrictions.

For seniors, adopting a growth mindset can be truly transformative. It is never too late to make healthy changes, and having this perspective can help you negotiate the problems that typically accompany aging, such as managing sciatica pain. It encourages us to view problems as chances for personal growth, to view defeats as transient, and to keep an insatiable quest for knowledge. However, the advantages do not end there.

A growth mindset can benefit your physical health by motivating you to exercise consistently and make healthier lifestyle choices. It boosts your emotional resilience and well-being while decreasing stress and anxiety. It also promotes a cheerful attitude, which can lead to better connections with family and friends, one of the biggest treasures in our golden years.

Remember, it's as simple as:

- Embracing challenges: Instead of seeing challenges as roadblocks, view them as opportunities to learn and grow. Approach them with curiosity and an open mind.
- The power of "yet": Whenever you catch yourself saying, "I can't do this," add the word "yet" at the end. It opens the door to future growth, self-belief, motivation, and confidence.
- Love learning: Commit to lifelong learning. Whether it's reading a book, picking up a new hobby, or exploring pain relief techniques, keep your mind engaged.
- Surrounding yourself with positivity: Seek out positive influences and surround yourself with people who support your growth mindset and your pain-free journey.

A growth mindset also allows you to take control of your health and well-being well into your senior years. Then there's the dynamic combination that can take your journey to the next level: a nutritious diet along with regular exercise.

These two components are more than just partners; they are the antidotes to sciatica pain reduction and total well-being. A good diet gives your body the fuel it needs to power through activity and recuperate quickly. It ensures that your body can not only execute but also recover from exercises, which is very crucial for seniors suffering from sciatica pain.

Also, we have looked into the importance of maintaining a healthy weight when it comes to managing sciatica, and being active burns those unwanted calories while a balanced diet maintains your ideal weight.

The combination of exercise and a healthy diet is great for encouraging and establishing a healthy routine and reinforcing accountability. You can plan your meals and workouts together, further fuelling consistency in both areas. Regular exercise revs up your metabolism aids in appetite control, and improves sleep quality, all of which are essential for pain management and overall well-being.

Exercise, particularly low-impact activities, can enhance joint health and flexibility, reducing inflammation and pain. You see the perfect combination. Your mental well-being also benefits from exercise, as it releases endorphins that improve mood and reduce stress. Plus, exercise and a healthy diet together minimize the risk of chronic diseases commonly associated with aging.

It's important to remember that choosing the right exercises to suit your needs and abilities is crucial. Opt for workouts that address your specific limitations, are sustainable and enjoyable, and focus on sciatica pain relief.

Remember, consistency is more important than intensity for seniors. Quality over quantity. Be mindful during your workouts, focusing on every breath and every movement. Rest and recovery are the cornerstones of your routine. Be sure to never skimp on these aspects.

Lastly, when it comes to fitness, make wise choices that align with your lifestyle and limitations. Remember the value of mental health, social connection, and a good view of life. The path does not end here; it is a continuous dedication to your health and well-being. Strength is the foundation for vitality and freedom on the canvas of life. We learn from sciatica that each minute is an opportunity to rise above pain and appreciate the gift of living fully in our older years.

So, take that first step, stay committed, and reap the rewards of a pain-free and enjoyable senior life. You've got this!

Without your voice we don't exist.
Please, support us and
<u>leave a honest review</u>
<u>on Amazon</u>

Just scan this QR code with your phone's camera and leave a review

Printed in Great Britain
by Amazon